# PRAISE FOR CALVIN NOWELL

"Wow! This book is amazing. It will change your life from the inside out. Calvin's transparency is used by God to make you laugh and make you cry to bring about real change and real deliverance. I believe if you read this book with an open heart, everlasting change will take place."
—CECE WINANS, *recording artist*

"Calvin Nowell is an amazingly talented individual and just a great person. His resolve to lose weight, and his follow-through, is an inspiration to all of us who know him. As a matter of fact, Calvin has become a great inspiration to many people who have never met him but know of his tremendous accomplishment. I'm proud of Calvin and grateful for his friendship."
—MICHAEL W. SMITH, *recording artist*

"I have had the opportunity to work with Calvin on multiple levels and have always been impressed by his integrity. Not only is he a talented musician, but he is also a great communicator with a powerful story to tell."
—TOBYMAC, *recording artist*

"I have seen Calvin make tremendous progress over the years. He looks totally different than when I first met him. He is not only different physically, but emotionally and spiritually. . . . Losing weight is not just a physical challenge, but an emotional and spiritual as well, and that is what Calvin can help you accomplish."
—ALLAN HOUSTON, *former NBA player (New York Knicks)*

"I've heard Calvin sing live many times. His vocals and music are inspiring; his ministry is unique."
—MICHAEL MCDONALD, *recording artist*

"Sometimes being a professional musician can breed a level of cynicism. Then there comes along an artist like Calvin Nowell who immediately and all at once restores your hope for the future of music and transforms you into a die-hard fan. 'Truth' and 'Start Somewhere' have impacted me deeply and, I am convinced, permanently. So far Calvin is the only 'unknown' artist in heavy—make that constant—rotation on my mp3 player. . . . Our family got the most pleasant surprise blessing when this unfamiliar and unassuming young guest stood to lead worship one Sunday. Little did we know that we would be 'airlifted' into the holy place of worship of the Most High before we could say, 'Who is Calvin Nowell?' We haven't been the same since."
—KIRK WHALUM, *jazz recording artist*

"Calvin has a one-of-a-kind talent and a heart to match it. His life and testimony are inspirational to everyone he encounters. He has sung with me on several occasions, and I am always inclined to give him the lead mic—he's that good! I love his voice, I love his story . . . and so will you!"
—NICOLE C. MULLEN, *recording artist*

"If a trumpet could speak and sing, it would sound like Calvin Nowell—clear, distinct, and compelling. This soul brother is a spirit man—he goes right to the heart and lifts you into the presence of God."
—JAMES RYLE, *speaker, author, and founding board member of Promise Keepers*

"A powerful and passionate artist whose life and voice embody the message of strength in humility."
—MARK HEIMERMANN, *Dove Award–winning producer (DC Talk, Michael W. Smith, Amy Grant)*

"Calvin is a living testimony of total surrender to the lordship of Jesus Christ. I am honored to call him my friend. He's an inspiration to my family, to our ministry, and to me personally. His talent is evident. His music will minister to and inspire people from every walk of life. But his heart for worship and leading others is more than words can describe. . . . His personal story of weight loss has impacted me in a unique way. I've heard others' stories but never this close to home. His biblical and practical approach to weight loss will inspire anyone who is willing to surrender and fight."
—JOE KATINA OF THE KATINAS

"Calvin's testimony has had a profound impact on so many lives, not only because of the visible transformation that he went through, but more importantly because of his ability to address deeper issues that we all deal with. His powerful testimony complements his ministry through music in a very natural way. He is a gifted young man, and I am sure many will be blessed by what God is doing through him."
—JAMES KATINA OF THE KATINAS

*start* **SOMEWHERE**

# *start* SOMEWHERE

## CALVIN NOWELL
### with GAYLA ZOZ

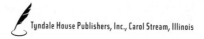
Tyndale House Publishers, Inc., Carol Stream, Illinois

Visit Tyndale's exciting Web site at www.tyndale.com.

*TYNDALE* and Tyndale's quill logo are registered trademarks of Tyndale House Publishers, Inc.

*Start Somewhere: Losing What's Weighing You Down from the Inside Out*

Designed by Jessie McGrath

Published in association with the literary agency of Stoner & Associates, P.O. Box 1074, Brentwood, TN 37024.

Scripture quotations are taken from the *Holy Bible*, New Living Translation, copyright © 1996, 2004, 2007 by Tyndale House Foundation. Used by permission of Tyndale House Publishers, Inc., Carol Stream, Illinois 60188. All rights reserved.

**Library of Congress Cataloging-in-Publication Data**

Nowell, Calvin.
   Start somewhere : losing what's weighing you down from the inside out / Calvin Nowell, with Gayla Zoz.
      p. cm.
   ISBN 978-1-4143-2331-2 (sc)
   1. Habit breaking—Religious aspects—Christianity. 2. Liberty—Religious aspects—Christianity. 3. Self-defeating behavior. 4. Weight loss—Religious aspects—Christianity. 5. Nowell, Calvin. I. Zoz, Gayla. II. Title.
BV4598.7.N69 2009
248.4—dc22                                                          2009022888

Printed in the United States of America

15   14   13   12   11   10   09
 7    6    5    4    3    2    1

*To my mother, Cordelia Nowell*

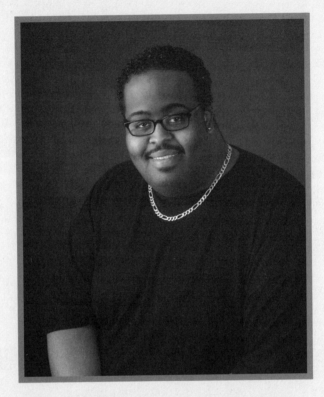

▶ *This is where my journey from 475 pounds began. . . .*

# CONTENTS

# ACKNOWLEDGMENTS

I WOULD LIKE TO EXTEND personal thanks to all the readers who have purchased this book. It is my prayer that this journey will encourage you to become the best you can be.

To my Creator and Savior, Jesus Christ: thank you for life and for turning my misery into my motivation.

Mom, I dedicate this book to you. My eyes are watering as I think about all the prayers and support you have shown me from birth to manhood. I love you so much, and I am glad that you are able to witness the promises of God within me. Dad, thanks for always providing for me and for making me who I am. I appreciate how you have helped so many deal with the struggles of life throughout the years. I believe that I am able to do the same because of your example.

To my sister Lynette, thanks for always being the best sister and supporting my career and aspirations throughout the years. Love ya. To my other sisters, Joy and Chloe: "Stay with it." You have always been my little sisters and have supported me throughout the years. I love you both, and I pray that I can be a blessing to you in the future with your dreams. To my nieces, Kristen and Lauren, you make me the proudest uncle. I am so happy about the women you both have turned out to be. Stay focused and determined.

To my pastor, Steve Berger, I can't even begin to put into words what you and your family mean to me. You have been the best spiritual father, mentor, brother, friend, and walking buddy. Thanks for helping me achieve my dreams musically and spiritually. Grace Chapel is the best church I have ever been a part of ("Put on your seat belt . . . and buckle up!").

To my best friend, Keenan. Thanks for standing in the trenches with me since tenth grade. You are the brother I never had, and you have been truly selfless in supporting me. Love you, bro. To my other bro, B. Reith. Thanks for fighting through life's challenges with me. You have been an amazing brother and accountability partner. Also, I am honored to be able to manage your career. You are going to make me rich one day.

To Sal Oliveri, you have been another rock in my journey. Thanks for contributing to my music. I am excited about working with you on many other projects. To Leanne Palmore, thanks for all your spiritual encouragement and many funny phrases now known throughout America.

To all my other great friends, Aaron Rudd, Donnie Gillespie, Walt Smith, Tommy and Wanda Dove, John Gray, Eric Lige, and James Katina, thank you.

To my great band and singers, thanks for supporting my testimony while on the road. Love all of you. To every church that believed in me and allowed me to share with your congregation, thank you very much. To all my other friends and family, thank you. I am afraid I may be leaving some folks out; however, please know that my heart is thanking you.

To Phil Stoner, thanks for helping me birth this book. You are the best agent. This would not be possible without you. To Gayla Zoz, I can't even begin to tell you how much you strengthened this book. This was by far the easiest collaboration. Last but not least, thanks to the staff at Tyndale House Publishers for your belief in my story. Thank you, Nancy Clausen, for your strong belief. Thank you for sticking with me and not giving up on me. I pray that this book goes above and beyond your expectations.

# CHAPTER 1

# THE LONG ROAD TO SIZE 66

How do you get to be 475 pounds?

The same way you get to be 10, 30, 50, or 100 pounds overweight. One bite at a time.

Unwrap, bite, chew, savor, swallow. Repeat.

The road to bigness is the same for most of us. Ahead is the hope that tomorrow will be different. Out there shimmering on the horizon is the next diet and the certainty that life will be perfect when you lose that weight. Behind you is a road littered with broken promises and diet failures—or in my case, burger wrappers, supersize fry boxes, all-you-can-eat buffet receipts, and the shiny little papers used to pick up doughnuts.

No one gets fat without secrets. And I had plenty.

### The Early Years—Secret Shame

If you're looking for a dramatic backstory, you won't find it here. There wasn't anything shocking about my upbringing. I was an average kid growing up in an average family in an average city in the middle of America. My sister and I were raised in a stable two-parent home. Mom worked as a secretary at the EPA. Dad worked as a truck driver. Mom prayed a lot. Dad swore a lot. Mom's goal was to raise me to be a spiritual person, rooted in the Bible. Dad's goal was to raise me to be a man who could hold down a job with benefits.

Have you ever felt that you were switched at birth—that maybe in the hospital where you were born members of a royal family were giving birth at the same time, and somehow you were their baby and ended up getting sent home with the wrong family? From as early as I can remember, that's how I felt. I was in the wrong place, in the wrong time, in the wrong body. I was more sensitive than everybody else. My head was bigger than other kids' heads. My body was sturdy and thick, not wisp thin like my friends'. I was afraid of everything—of dogs, of other people, of swimming, of spending the night away from home, of mean people. I never told anyone about my fears. They were my secrets.

Bullies were everywhere, waiting to pounce. The earliest ones were family members. When I was six, my older cousins pressured me to fight another boy in the neighborhood to see who would win. I was petrified.

Fast-forward a few years to the playground, where the older kids made fun of my head. "Here comes rock head," they taunted. "Hey, big head! Boy, your head is huge. Look at his head."

When you're ten years old, what do you do with comments like that? Put your head on a diet? You laugh along and pretend that it doesn't bother you, when in reality the shame feels like the hot iron used to brand a cow—only you're being branded a freak. As you sidle away, hearing the snickers, seeing the people snort and point, you laugh along, trying to act like you're in on the joke instead of *being* the joke.

I always thought I was big, although my body was actually pretty normal for a kid. Up until about the seventh grade, no one would have called me fat. I was an active, healthy, solid kid who just happened to need husky-size pants. That husky label was a secret shame for me. Normal kids didn't wear husky jeans. So I figured I must be fat.

If I couldn't get acceptance from being a normal-size person, I decided to get it from being really, really good at something else. Soccer was my first attempt. I was just an average player, and my fire-breathing coach screamed at me all the time. I hated it. And because my parents never attended my practices like the other parents did, they never saw what was happening. I watched as the other parents got in the coach's face when he yelled at their kids. Where were my parents?

Okay, before we go any further, let me just clarify one thing. If you're reading this thinking, *Oh no, not another dysfunctional adult blaming his parents for his irresponsible, out-of-control behavior,* while rolling your eyes, I'll issue the standard disclaimer. Yes, my parents did the best they could with what they had. Things weren't easy for them, and they were raising me the way they were raised.

But at the time, my immature brain truly believed that things might be different if my parents were more encouraging and more affirming. I couldn't help thinking that things would be better for me if my mom and dad were more like my friends' parents, who showed up at games and were involved in their lives. Other kids had dads who said they loved them. Other kids had parents who listened to the same music. Other kids had parents who were cool. Why couldn't mine be more like that?

End of rant. I promise that I will take responsibility for my own behavior. It just doesn't happen in this chapter.

When I quit soccer, my dad's reaction was harsh. "What's wrong with you?" he yelled, reminding me that if I didn't stay in sports, I would end up like he had been: 100 pounds overweight and destined for a lifelong battle of the bulge. I was too young to understand that he was simply trying to spare me the ridicule and shame that he had experienced while facing the world as a fat man. I only saw a dad who seemed to have been born without a shred of empathy.

Next I tried basketball. My seventh-grade tryout involved a scrimmage with a team of horrible players who weren't even good enough to pass me the ball so I could show what I could do. I didn't make the team and told myself I would try again next year. Things didn't go so well then, either. I broke my hand two weeks before tryouts, which meant I wouldn't make the eighth-grade team. There was no way I would play in high school.

When it was clear that my dreams of athletic greatness weren't going to materialize, I gave up on sports. My overeating shifted into overdrive, and the weight piled on.

## From Rock Head to Big Cal

How do you get to be 475 pounds without anyone seeing you eat?

It can be done. Trust me, I know.

Secret eating is pretty common for a lot of fat people. It was for me, too, starting in the eighth grade. But it never occurred to me that I was hiding. At the time, it just seemed normal.

Growing up, I was always told to finish all the food on my plate. There was never any emphasis on good or bad foods.

There were no discussions about healthy eating. There was just a plate in front of me and the expectation that I would eat it all. So I did.

But I always wanted more. Intuitively I knew that the amounts I wanted weren't normal, and I realized that in order to get as much as I wanted, I would have to find a way to eat it in secret. By the middle of my eighth-grade year, I had become a master of sneak eating. I would pig out before my mom got home from work, and then I would act like I hadn't eaten anything and enjoy a hearty dinner with the family.

No one might have seen me eat, but everyone could see my growing girth. By the ninth grade, I was in a size 38, but I could still buy clothes from the regular store. By my sophomore year, I had crossed the threshold into a size 42 and officially entered the "big and tall" universe. But even so, I told myself that I still looked good, and I went to great lengths to hide my weight with my clothing choices. I scouted out the latest trends in the fashion-forward men's stores and then searched for those same styles in the big and tall store. Sometimes I could find them; sometimes I couldn't.

Food became my best friend. Eating was the one thing that soothed the sting and shame of failing at sports. There is no better listener in this world than a chocolate cake. Food never made any demands. I could turn to food no matter what—to celebrate with, to complain to, to be soothed by. It never asked for anything in return.

Sneaking, lying, and stealing became the norm. Whenever there was a birthday in our family, we had a cake. I always took my piece during the celebration, all the while silently plotting how I could get more. The next day after school, I would eat the rest of the cake and then tell my mother that friends stopped by and ate it with me. I would bake cakes, cookies, and brownies, claiming I was making them for school, and then hide them in my room and eat them all myself.

The bigger I got, the more my dad nagged me to lose weight. "When you get older, you won't be able to find a job," he shouted. "You're never going to be able to support yourself— or your family!" The more he yelled, the more I ate. I grew and grew. No one was calling me "rock head" anymore. Now they were calling me Big Cal. Or was it Big Cow? I was never sure.

When I turned sixteen, the game changed. Up to this point, my eating had been limited to what I could bake, make, or steal from the house. But with a driver's license, a working car, and gas money, there were no limits. I could drive to the places that sold all my favorite foods. Even better, I now had a place to eat, far from the prying eyes of my parents. My car was my personal binge-mobile. It was just me, the food, the wrappers, and the nearest commercial Dumpster where I would get rid of the evidence.

I ate whatever I wanted. If one was good, two were better— and dozens were ideal. My meals were huge. I always had at least two helpings of the entrée, and usually more. I snacked constantly. I ate whenever I was hungry. If we didn't have what I wanted in the house, I went to get it. If I didn't have money, I stole change from my parents. I even spent the two-dollar coins in my dad's collection—always a little at a time so he wouldn't notice.

People might know that I was big, I told myself, but no one thought I was obese. Obese people were sloppy-big with giant guts that my friends called front booties. Obese people looked bad. Sometimes they even smelled bad. They weren't stylish or cool. I was stylish *and* cool. I was a big guy who carried his weight well. I might have been fat, but I still looked cool.

Looking cool and being accepted by the in crowd were extremely important to me. I dressed like I had money, believing that I could hide the consequences of my eating with clothes. If you wear a stylish jacket and great shoes, others will be so dazzled by your outfit that it won't dawn on them that you're the size of a double-wide, right? That's what Big Cal thought.

I wasn't a sports star, but I befriended the basketball stars, basking in their reflected glory and earning their approval by whipping the crowd into a frenzy on game nights. I was on the fringes of the in crowd, which meant interacting with in-crowd girls. There were five in particular I liked, but none of them liked me. "Calvin, you're like my brother," they would say, while I was screaming inside, *I don't want to be your brother—I want to be your man!*

My secret fear was that I wasn't cool at all. And there was plenty of evidence to support this. I wasn't the best at anything, though I tried a lot of things. I played in the band until junior year. I ran for student body president and homecoming king and lost. More than anything, I wanted acceptance, praise, and encouragement. But it never came. I did like to sing, but I didn't feel comfortable with my gift. I was afraid to tell my family that I liked to sing and never dared sing around them. It seemed I would never find my place.

So I ate.

## Size 54 in the Gang Showers

By the end of high school, my body bore the scars of years of unrestrained eating. I was covered with stretch marks. Having a girlfriend was out of the question. I knew that thin girls would never want to date an overweight guy like me because their friends would make fun of them. I consoled myself with the thought that my size was God's way of keeping me pure.

Being fat even influenced my choice of a college, since I was afraid of the community showers in the dorm. Clothes could hide the reality of my condition, but gang showers would reveal it to everyone. As a size 54, there was no way I was going to undress in front of anyone.

I figured I would go to Wright State University in Dayton, which was less than an hour from home. When I had visited there, I was elated to discover that each room shared a bathroom with an adjoining room. That sealed the deal. No one would have to see me naked. I applied and was accepted.

But my mother had other plans. "Why don't you apply to the University of Cincinnati," she suggested. Her reasons made sense. UC offered scholarships for minorities. But that would mean living at home and going to school as a commuter. Even though all the cool kids were going away to school, I applied to UC to please my mom. When I was offered a full scholarship and heard her praising God, I knew my decision was made. I went to UC, lived at home during my freshman year, and got an apartment near campus before my sophomore year.

Living on my own marked the end of my amateur status as an overeater. I spent every waking moment thinking about the next meal or snack, planning how to get it, eating the food in secret, getting rid of the evidence, and then looking forward to the next snack. Fast food was my favorite.

My college education involved more than just studying marketing and business. I perfected the art of stealth eating, and my strategies to avoid detection got more sophisticated. I would walk into the bakery and request a dozen doughnuts like I was ordering for several people.

"I think they want this, this, and this . . . with a bit of that," I would say, pointing out all my favorites and praying that the server didn't suspect I was going to eat them all myself.

I always volunteered to be the carryout courier for meals with my friends. I would order an extra meal, eat it in the car, throw away the evidence, and then eat my second dinner with the others.

I often went to Shoney's breakfast buffet alone and ate mountains of grits, eggs, sausages, hash browns, and more. And who could possibly be satisfied with one trip to the breakfast buffet? Two trips was my minimum. But when you're my size, you can't just go up again and again and not expect dirty looks. So I went in with a plan. On my first trip to the buffet, I carefully monitored who was in the restaurant. I then delayed the second trip until the patrons had been replaced with new ones. I didn't want the same set of people to see me on my second trip, which was always timed so that the new people would think I was going for the first time. I was very concerned about what people thought, and I didn't want the other diners to think I was a pig. My worst fear was that someone would come over to my table and stand there like the buffet police, hands on hips, frowning down at me and saying, "You're the size of a house, and you've been up there three times. Come on, man, leave some for the rest of us!" I was terrified of the rejection that I always felt was just around the corner. It never occurred to me that the servers might be drawing their own conclusions. A 400-pound guy lurking in the restaurant—what would *you* think he was doing?

Because of this, I found it easier to eat privately, away from others. No matter where I was, no matter what happened to me, food was a reliable, legal sedative that kept me securely insulated from the realities of life—and my potential.

## A Life in between Bites

By now, you may be thinking that all I did was eat. It's true that a great amount of time was spent chewing. But in between bites, things were happening for me during those years.

In between bites, I discovered I could sing. I had never been in church or school choirs when I was growing up, but I had always loved music. My friend Chloe joined the UC gospel choir and invited me to do the same. So I did, and I loved it. The other singers became like family to me, and everyone told me what a great tenor I was. That meant a lot to me, and it made me want to sing more.

Members of the choir encouraged me to enter the Mr. and Ms. African American arts festival competition. In my mind I thought, *Yeah, but I'm fat.* The encouragement I heard, however, was a rare treat for me, and I took the plunge. I desperately wanted to be accepted.

For the talent portion of the competition, I sang "Running Back to You" by gospel singer Fred Hammond. My family was sitting in the audience that day, and it was the first time they had ever heard me attempt a solo. They were absolutely floored. *Calvin can sing! Wow!* I ended up winning the talent competition. Although it wasn't enough to win the honor of Mr. African American, it planted a seed in my mind. Maybe I did have a gift. Maybe it was music. When the gospel choir director began giving me little solo parts, I knew I had finally found my niche.

In between bites, I discovered the Lord. A UC football player, Hassan Champion, invited me to a Bible study he was leading. A bunch of us guys would pile into his room and dig into the Scripture. I began to take spiritual things much more seriously.

Up to that point, I had gone to church mainly out of habit or to meet other people my age. Now I became serious about the real point of meeting with God. I had been introduced to the Lord as a child at the small charismatic church my family attended. I had always questioned the authenticity of religion and faith, however, because it seemed to me that worship was more about high drama and emotion than real-life practice. Even so, my parents raised me to be sensitive toward the things of God. Whenever I was rejected at school, my mother always encouraged me to turn to the Lord. Now I began to realize that faith could—and should—be proactive as well as reactive.

Hassan often approached me and said things like, "Man, I was thinking about you the other day, and this Scripture came into my mind." Then he'd quote a verse that seemed especially applicable to something that was going on in my life at the time.

"I want to encourage you that God wants to do great things in your life," he would tell me. That really made an impact on me, and as a result, I began reading the Bible more intentionally. I surrounded myself with spiritual friends, joined Lincoln Heights Baptist Church, and began singing in the choir.

Unfortunately my newly discovered faith did nothing to lessen the intensity of my binges. Somehow it never occurred to me to hand over my eating problem to the Lord.

In between bites, I entered the job market. It was 1998. I had a freshly minted bachelor's degree and an impressive résumé— which included numerous summer internships and extracurricular activities—that landed me a number of interviews.

Employers were always quite interested—until they met me in person. Was it my weight? Certainly, seeing a candidate walk in wearing a size 56 or 58 suit had to be a jolt. But was I really so big that employers wouldn't want me, despite my skills?

One day I summoned the courage to get on my sister's digital scale. It said 426. My first thought was, *No way this is right. The scale is broken. There's no way I'm over 400 pounds. It has to be a mistake.* My father's warnings about being overweight and out of work rang through my head, but I put those thoughts out of my mind and kept looking for a job.

A friend of mine, John Gray, organized gospel musicals for live theater, and he invited me to join him in a play being produced in Pittsburgh. I'd never done that kind of thing before—I wasn't sure I could. But John seemed to think my voice was right for it, so I said I'd try. I ended up spending ten months in Pittsburgh working on the production. I sang onstage, and I also put my marketing degree to good use during the daytime, running promotions for the show and handling other offstage work. I loved it. But the joy of using my talents wasn't enough to distract me from my first love: food.

Unlike many overweight people, yo-yo dieting had not been a part of my history. Though I had never really given dieting a serious try, it did occur to me that I might need to lose a few pounds if I ever wanted to get a stable job. So I tried the Atkins diet while I was living in Pittsburgh. I could tell that my clothes were fitting a little looser, but I threw in the towel after just a month when I tried to weigh myself and couldn't find a scale big enough to hold me.

In 1999, after the play had run its course, John and I had dinner with the senior pastor of a vibrant church in Pittsburgh.

"I hear the Lord saying you desire mentors," the senior

pastor said to me, "someone to show you the way." I was blown away. How could he see into my heart? How did he know that I had always been looking for encouragement? It was prophetic. I decided to stay in Pittsburgh in order to take a job in his church. His teaching was incredible; I had never heard anything about growing in Christ that made so much sense.

The pay wasn't much, but it worked for me. The elders said they really wanted to mentor young men and help them become all God wanted them to be. But it didn't take long to find out what kind of "mentoring" they had in mind. An elder said to me one day, "Calvin, I would like to talk to you about some of the issues in your life, including your weight." *Don't go there,* I thought, while toying with the idea of a trip to McDonald's. Although the elders were right, it really bothered me that they were only looking at my weaknesses, with no regard to my strengths. I simply was not yet ready to deal with my weight.

Eventually, after months of working seventy-hour weeks serving seven different elders with competing demands and making a paltry eight hundred dollars a month, I gathered the courage to ask for a raise. The elders had other ideas—I was laid off due to the "budget crunch." I thought my life was over.

At the end of 2000, still reeling from the rejection of losing my job, I looked around my bare high-rise apartment. With little more than a bed and a grocery cart to hold my belongings, I asked God once again where I truly belonged. By this point, two years of my life had gone by since I had graduated from college. I had a degree and experience, yet my world was in chaos. I didn't see the point of living.

I opened my Bible and read the story about Elijah feeling discouraged on Mount Sinai. I could certainly identify. God eventually spoke to him through "a gentle whisper" (1 Kings 19:12).

I prayed in that moment, *Lord, I sure wish You'd whisper something to me.* Then I turned out the light and went to sleep.

The phone rang, startling me. I fumbled in the dark for the receiver and mumbled a dull "Hello?"

It was John Gray, on tour somewhere. He wasted no time with pleasant greetings, instead stunning me with a declaration: "Man, you need to move to Nashville!"

"Nashville? What? Why would I do that?"

"It's where all the music stuff happens, man. You've got a gift. You need to put it in a place where it can really grow. I'm serious!"

I told him I would think about it. When I hung up the phone, I had to admit I didn't have any better ideas. By the next day, I had decided to follow John's bold directive. Could this be my chance for a new beginning?

## Pushing 60 in Music City

When I arrived in Nashville in 2002, there was less and less time in between bites. I didn't know what I weighed, but I knew I was big. I had ballooned up to a size 60. But I wasn't going to let something as silly as a number get between me and my dream of being in the music business. I didn't have enough confidence in my vocal abilities to think I could become a recording artist, so I thought I would go through the back door and learn everything I could about the industry.

Nashville offered plenty of options, as John Gray had said. A friend of mine, LeAnne Palmore, was a backup singer for Michael W. Smith and CeCe Winans. Michael was working on a worship DVD in Canada, and they were having a hard time finding a male tenor. LeAnne called me to see if I was available.

Of course I was available! Although I jumped at the chance, LeAnne knew me well enough to know that I was not fully confident. She said to me, "Calvin, you've got to be *on it*." In other words, this was a big deal. I had to work hard and take it seriously. And I did.

Singing with Michael was a life-changing experience for me. I could see so much opportunity in front of me as a full-time musician. But would any of it really come to pass?

I settled into a predominantly white church, Oasis Worship Centre, where Pastor Danny Chambers welcomed me warmly and even invited me to lead worship at one midweek service. The presence of the Lord seemed to come down that night. People were swept up in praise. More opportunities came along, and soon I was on the staff as worship pastor while I worked on my music career. I loved being a worship pastor, but I also wanted to explore every opportunity available to me in the music industry.

Even though my life seemed to be going in the right direction, I was struggling with my weight. I was approaching the upper end of what big and tall stores carried. They didn't go beyond a 60-inch waist or 6X in the casual lines. I was getting bigger. What was I going to do for clothes in the future? Would I have to hire a custom tailor? Would I be reduced to getting clothes from a catalog? Would this mean the end of looking cool?

I dreaded flying. After shoehorning myself into the aisle seat on a jam-packed red-eye from LA to Nashville, I knew that the woman in the seat next to me was not happy about the situation. I spent the five-hour flight in her airspace. Her resentment felt like darts.

I had a hard time getting in and out of cars. The steering wheel was always too close to my stomach. I dreaded having people watch me try to squeeze in.

I even found sitting down to be an adventure. Would the chair hold, or would it break? I could never be sure. I was humiliated when I sat on a friend's bed and bent the metal frame. "Oh, that's okay," he said, careful to hide his embarrassment. But his sidelong glances told me that it wasn't okay. Most of all, *I* knew it wasn't okay.

Over the Thanksgiving holiday in 2002, I returned to Ohio to sing at a friend's wedding. I was wearing a size 64 long coat and size 60 pants. The rented tuxedo jacket was the biggest they had. It was so tight around my middle that I couldn't button it. I really needed the next size up. *The next jacket you buy will be a 66,* I told myself. *This is ridiculous.*

A few days before heading back to Cincinnati for Christmas, I had chest pains. Heart attacks ran in my family. *You need to do something,* I told myself. I hadn't had insurance since college. I never went to the doctor. I sometimes took my blood pressure in the grocery store, and it was always fine. *I'm big, but I'm healthy,* I rationalized.

But now I was scared. I had lost my job at the church due to "financial difficulties" and was unemployed again. Nothing was changing. Except my size. I was still eating, still hiding, and still getting bigger by the second. It takes a lot of food to maintain a weight as high as mine had become.

My story was going to end soon if I didn't do something. It was just a matter of how it ended. I didn't have the courage to commit suicide. But it was clear that I was perfectly capable of eating myself to death.

My options: die fast or die slow.

Or be open to change.

Something about the chest pains and the loneliness and the too-tight suit jacket and the prospect of shopping from a catalog pushed me over the edge. Standing at the intersection of desperation and willingness, I was too big to keep eating and too scared to stop. I had crossed the line from big to obese. My best efforts had landed me squarely where my father always said I would be: fat, unemployed, broke, and destined for an early death. My father's nightmare had become my own.

Maybe it was time to be open to change.

The only question was where to begin.

CHAPTER **2**

# WEIGHT COMES IN MANY SHAPES

I HAD TO START SOMEWHERE.

The road to somewhere started in Cincinnati. It was December 2002. My friend LeAnne and I were at a Christmas party at the home of a wealthy acquaintance in Nashville, and we ended up singing some songs for the crowd.

Our host was impressed by our performance. "Man, you really need to do something," he said. "I've got the money if you've got the time."

Inside I was giddy. Could his comments be the Lord's way of saying that my dreams of a music career could really come true?

Despite his affirmation, my initial excitement was overshadowed by doubts: I was out of work, fatter than ever, and worried about the stabbing pains in my chest. It seemed too good to be true. After all, things like that just didn't work out for me.

I spent Christmas in Cincinnati with my family, and before

heading back to Nashville, I went to a worship service at my home church. Before the service began, the associate minister began his message with this: "I don't know what it is, but I keep seeing dimes everywhere I go. I've been seeing them all week. Even on the way into the building today I saw at least ten dimes. I'm not even trying to be superspiritual about it. I just think the Lord is going to say something to us by the end of the service."

I was sitting in the back of the church feeling sorry for myself when the senior pastor pointed at me and said, "Calvin, why don't you come up here and share what's going on in Nashville." I didn't want to admit that not much was going on for me in Nashville, so I told them all about my encounter with the millionaire. I knew that it should have been a bright spot in my otherwise cloudy existence, but I was having trouble seeing it that way.

The pastor had other ideas. "That's the Lord," he said as I returned to my seat. "It's prophetic. God is saying that if you're willing to do what you need to do, He's got the provision for you."

And that's when it hit me. My associate pastor hadn't been seeing dimes; he was seeing *change*. He was picking up change. A little bit here. A little bit there.

And then it *really* hit me.

When you pick up small change, you end up with big change. If you're flat broke and you find a dime, you now have ten cents more than what you had before. Let's say you find ten dimes a day. That adds up to a dollar a day. At the end of a week you have seven dollars, and at the end of the month it's now twenty-eight dollars. It was a profound insight to me at the time.

## Picking Up Change

Why had I never seriously attempted to diet before? Because I felt like I had to do it all at once. The thought of making wholesale changes in my lifestyle just seemed too overwhelming, especially when I had so much weight to lose.

It doesn't help that we live in a culture that tells us we're not advancing unless we make quantum leaps. If I found a dollar in change, I used to think, *Man, it's only a dollar. I'm still broke— I'm not blessed.* But in that worship service, God showed me that picking up a little change each day would add up to a significant difference in my life over time. I had always thought if something didn't happen instantly, it wasn't worth doing. On some level, I expected to come to the altar and have God remove all 200 pounds at one time.

I had believed I was stuck. But was I really? I knew I had to lose weight. I knew I couldn't tackle everything all at once. But I *could* start somewhere by making one tiny change. And one change might lead to another. That initial tiny change could mean the beginning of a process that might eventually result in big change.

Picking up change became my motto for 2003.

During my drive home to Nashville, I called a trainer friend and said, "I'm ready to do it. This is a new year, and I'm picking up change. I'm going to try it."

When my trainer asked for a ninety-day commitment, I was skeptical but agreed. If you sow a season of your life, then you'll reap a lifestyle, he told me. So right there, in the car on the road to Nashville, I committed to giving ninety days to my trainer. I was ready to try another way, taking teeny-tiny steps and picking up change along the way.

And then a Scripture came into my head:

*At the name of Jesus every knee should bow, in heaven and on earth and under the earth, and every tongue confess that Jesus Christ is Lord, to the glory of God the Father.*
—PHILIPPIANS 2:10-11

It was almost as if I could hear God in heaven saying, "You can choose whatever god you want and you can do whatever you want to do, but the bottom line is that you all will bow to Me one day or another." It dawned on me that food had been my god for a long, long time. It was my comforter and my confessor. Now it was time to change.

## Resist to Expand

If you're on the edge of your seat waiting to see what amazing new miracle weight-loss fad I followed, you're going to be disappointed. I lost my weight through old-fashioned diet and exercise. I made small changes in my behavior that became habits.

The big news was that losing weight had less to do with what I put in my mouth than what was going on between my ears. As I began to work with my trainer, I could see that he was going to do more than just challenge me to eat differently and move more. He was going to help me look at things differently.

One early insight knocked me over. He explained that when you resist, you expand. No one understands this principle better than bodybuilders. They don't just endure the discomfort of lifting weights, they embrace it, knowing that their effort is going to pay off in a better physique.

Could the same principle apply to my spirit? If I resisted the urge to eat when faced with the struggles of my life, would I grow as a person? After flexing those spiritual muscles time and again, I might even eventually be able to surrender the crutch that food had always been in my life.

## Weight in Sin

My problem was, and always had been, the weight between my ears. I was ironing my clothes for church one day when the Lord whispered to me, *You may think this is about losing weight, but it's not about the pounds. It's about laying aside every weight in sin.*

Talk about a burning-bush moment! I nearly burned a hole in my shirt. The Lord had just issued my marching orders straight from Hebrews 12.

Weight can be defined as anything that impedes motion. It's anything that slows us down. Weight in sin is any burden or blockage that keeps us stuck, stumbling, and sick.

I wear my weight in sin on my body, making it obvious to everyone. But some weight isn't so visible; weight in sin wears many disguises. It often appears as a natural appetite spiraled out of control. For many, the out-of-control appetite is an activity like eating, smoking, racking up credit card debt, indulging in affairs, using drugs, or drinking. For others, it is a way of thinking, like pride, low self-esteem, vanity, or grandiosity.

If you . . .

> want to start doing something but won't
>
> want to stop doing something but can't
>
> hope to keep doing something but don't

. . . it's a safe bet that you're being crushed by weight in sin. Being fat isn't the half of it. Just as real are the weights of debt, lust, smoking, rejection, laziness, low self-esteem, broken relationships, alcohol, drugs, and other things that tie us down.

People who say that they don't have weight are lying—and maybe *lying* is their weight. Everyone is carrying something; we all have our baggage. I'll start by telling you what's in mine. You already know that food is an issue for me, but it's not the only one.

I really care about what people think of me. I guess you could say I'm one of those people with low self-esteem, and the thought that someone might not like me fills me with terror. I have always been a slave to the approval of others. I'm desperately afraid of disappointing people—of letting them down in any way.

As a person who has struggled with his weight all his life, I have seen this fear manifest itself in many ways. The idea of starting a diet scared me to death. If I went off my food plan for a few days and gained a few pounds, I knew I would feel like a failure. Panic would set in, and I'd once again find myself in the cycle of perfectionism, where every slip leads to self-hatred, and self-hatred leads to a binge, and the binge leads to the promise uttered by dieters everywhere: "I'll start again on Monday."

If food issues are your "weight," this cycle may sound familiar. You slip up, and you feel like garbage. You're certain that everyone knows, that everyone is looking and judging, just waiting for you to screw up so they can roll their eyes and say smugly, "I knew he couldn't keep the weight off."

If you want to find out why you are overeating, stop overeating. Begin to ask yourself the question, "Why do I do what I do?" You'll get in touch with the real weight that's burdening your life. Even if you lose the pounds, you may find that you are forced to face the weight between your ears. That's what was happening with me. I could really feel the "food struggle" and the pain created by the way I perceived myself, others, and the world I lived in.

Maybe you can relate.

## Eight Steps to Freedom

There is no journey unless you make the decision to put down the remote control and get off the couch.

For me, the decision was simple. Once and for all, I decided to drop my weight in sin at the Lord's feet and let Him have all of me. That decision marked the beginning of my journey to freedom.

In the chapters ahead, you will see what happened after I made that critical decision. You will learn about a spiritual fitness program that works its magic in eight simple steps:

1. Own your own weight.
2. See God as your friend.
3. Take up a new perspective.
4. Get someone to hold you accountable.
5. Start somewhere.
6. Eliminate the excuses.
7. Accept the need for training wheels.
8. Persevere to the end.

These eight steps transformed my life, but they won't work for you unless you can say without reservation that you are done trying to fix yourself. These eight steps work best for people whose self-destructive behaviors have spiraled out of control and who have nowhere else to turn.

If you are desperate enough to let God into the dark recesses of your life, the next eight chapters show you what to do next.

Let us begin.

# CHAPTER 3

# STEP 1: OWN YOUR OWN WEIGHT

THE FIRST STEP to freedom is uncomfortable, because it calls us to name the specific burden that is limiting us. As diet counselors say, you have to own the number.

Owning the number forces you to come out of hiding. And hiding is one thing I did really well.

Looking back, it seems that I would do just about anything to avoid owning the number. If I didn't admit to myself how big I really was, then no one else would know either, right? It was like the peekaboo game, the one where a child covers his eyes and thinks others can't see him.

That was me—living in pure delusion. But that's where many of us live when we're burdened by a weight in sin that we haven't owned.

I had experienced this delusion in a big way in 2002, when I was close to my heaviest weight. My pastor's wife said, "We need the worship team to start dressing up, so Calvin, I'm taking you shopping!" I was horrified.

"No, no, no," I replied, trying not to sound desperate. "That's very sweet but so not necessary."

I knew that if I went shopping with her I would have to reveal that my shirt size was a 5X or a 6X. I was so focused on making sure no one else knew how big I was that I couldn't accept this generosity from a very loving woman.

My pastor's kindhearted wife would hear none of my protests. She went shopping without me and came back with a shirt. She was beaming when she handed it to me. "Oh, Calvin, this is so you!" I could imagine her holding it up in the store thinking, *Oh yeah. That's the one. It will fit for sure.*

It didn't. But I never told her.

I didn't want her to know how big I really was. I didn't want anyone to know.

But most of all, *I* didn't want to know. Because knowing would tell me what I was. Knowing that number would confirm my worst fear of all: that I had finally crossed the line from "just big" to "sloppy big" or, even worse, "smelly big."

This circle of delusion—wanting to manage what others thought of me so I could avoid facing the truth about myself— kept me imprisoned for years. Reality mattered far less than what I told myself others believed. *If you don't think I'm that big, then I'm not. Oh, and by the way, if you do think I'm that big, you're out of my life.*

I have always resisted knowing what *is*, but accepting reality shows what needs to be done.

## The Battle in the Brain

When your weight in sin is excess fat, the scale is a double-edged sword, and the battleground is in your head.

The scale is an important reality check. So is the measuring tape. But for many people with food issues, these simple tools of accountability take on a sinister new meaning. In the hands of the enemy, they become weapons of mass distraction that your brain uses to beat you up with unrealistic expectations about how things should be.

I had always hated the scale and was able to avoid it because no conventional scale would hold me. When I first started working with my trainer, he needed some way to check my progress. So he took my measurements.

When it was time for him to do the deed, the smooth feel of the tape measure around my middle brought up a sick feeling in my throat. I wanted the number to be 45 or 48 or even 50, but I knew it wouldn't be that low. I braced myself for my trainer's snickers. But they never came. Even with my 60-inch waist. Having someone else see the real truth about my size wasn't so terrible after all.

I gauged my progress by the measuring tape in the early days. And thank goodness I had it. If I hadn't seen the inches come off, I would have thrown in the towel after thirty days.

After several months, though, people started to notice a difference in my appearance. "Man, what's happening with you?" asked one friend who hadn't seen me in a while. "Are you losing weight?" It was great to hear the compliments, but the truth is I had no idea how much weight I had lost.

Eventually my trainer wanted to be able to monitor my progress with more than just the measuring tape. Six months into my weight-loss program, he told me to meet him at the YMCA. It was time to weigh in.

So there I was, in the buff in the men's locker room, getting ready to step on the scale and feeling a tremendous sense of dread. Was that the *Jaws* theme playing in the background?

What would the number be? It was killing me. I had been so good for so long. I was imagining what the number should be . . . I did the math—it should be about 280.

I stepped on the scale with my eyes closed, fully expecting the number to register well under 300 pounds.

When I opened my eyes, I gasped. Not only was my trainer pushing the little black bar past the 300 mark, he was going higher: 310, 320, 330. Doesn't holding your breath add at least 10 pounds? It must, because the number that day—after six months of diet and exercise—was 350!

Inside I was screaming. *Noooooooooooooooooo!*

I felt like a horrible person. I had failed. And so the three-way shouting match began.

> **Me to trainer:** I've been working so hard (sigh), and my weight is only just now what everyone thought it was when I first started (pout)!
>
> **Trainer to me:** Look at you! You're amazing. Can you see how far you've come?
>
> **Devil to me:** You're going nowhere. And did I mention that you're worthless?
>
> **Me to trainer:** But it's so little progress for so much work. It's supposed to be 280.
>
> **Trainer to me:** You've lost 12 inches in your waist! That's incredible progress!
>
> **Devil to me:** You still have a fat backside. Oh, and you're still ugly!
>
> **Me to trainer:** It's not happening fast enough.

**Trainer to me:** Don't get sucked in to the lie that you're failing, because you're not.

**Devil to trainer:** It's no lie. He ate so many doughnuts he's a cream stick with legs.

**Trainer to devil:** Remind Calvin of his past, and I'll remind you of your future!

Instead of savoring my progress, the only thing I could feel was anger. But the anger was rooted in something other than reality. I had been working so hard on this diet, and for what?

Ugh. It was terrible. I thought of quitting. *I might as well give up right now.* I was beating myself up because I didn't see the number I thought I should see. My expectations weren't met, and I was mad. The still, small voice in my heart was whispering, *Calvin, you might be expecting too much,* but it was being drowned out by the enemy's chest-thumping. I wanted to quit. And quitting was just another form of hiding.

## Hiding along the Way

I didn't quit. My trainer held me up—he kept encouraging me with support and affirmation. No one had ever encouraged me like that before. He made me want to continue; he made me want to be good to myself.

So I kept going. About a year into my journey, I was feeling positive about my progress. "Man, I'm good," I said to my trainer. "I've lost weight. I don't know if I need to do this anymore."

"All right," he said. "How about we take a picture of you naked and put it on the dashboard of your car? Look at it awhile, and then let me know if you still need my help."

Even then, after releasing around 100 pounds, I still wanted to quit. It's just that the desire to hide had morphed into something else. Now, instead of not wanting to own how big I was, I couldn't bear to face the shame. How could I have let myself go like this? How could I have let myself get so big in the first place?

Every time I got on the scale, I had those thoughts. Sometimes I became so obsessed with my failures that I couldn't see the successes I had made in the past year. At times I felt that it might be easier to avoid the scale altogether. The scale had become a torture device.

Like many dieters, I became obsessed with the number. If I stepped on the scale and liked the number I saw, I felt great. If not, I felt like a failure.

Thankfully my trainer helped me see that my expectations for myself were way out of line. On some level, I thought that I shouldn't have to deal with the same laws of thermodynamics that apply to everyone else. What do you mean, I can't lose 50 pounds by noon tomorrow? I've been sold a bill of goods!

It takes a lot of courage to face the reality of your own bad behavior when that behavior has consequences that everyone can see. I can't hide the consequences of my eating. I wear them. It takes even more courage to face the reality of bad behavior that others can't see, especially when those behaviors are done in secret.

It's just easier to hide.

## Honesty Brings Grace

It makes me think of Adam and Eve.

When the Lord said, "Where are you?" He already knew where Adam and Eve were. God already knew that they had broken His very simple rules. Maybe He was thinking, *Why not give them an opportunity to be honest? Let's see what they do.*

But they wouldn't be honest. They lied.

Adam could have said, "You know what, Lord? I did it. I ate the fruit that I knew I wasn't supposed to eat. I'm sorry." He could have owned up without any of the blame shifting or finger-pointing. But instead he hid. And later on his son Cain did the same thing.

God was angry. He didn't let Adam or Eve or Cain get away with hiding. I wonder if God might have been ready to extend grace to them if they hadn't tried to hide.

Grace is available to anyone who comes clean. In fact, He is just waiting for us to come clean.

## The Power of Coming Clean

God already knows the number . . .

> on the bathroom scale
>
> on the credit card statement
>
> of drinks you had
>
> of dollars you've spent on drugs
>
> of lies you've told to your spouse about where you were
>
> of times you've indulged in adultery

God already knows. So why not be honest?

What's happening in your life may be a lot like what happened in the Garden of Eden. You knew the rules, you screwed up, and now you're trying to hide from the consequences. Or you've allowed some natural appetite to spin out of control, and you can't stop it.

Maybe you're afraid to take your problems to your Creator. Maybe you don't tell the Lord what's going on because you're certain He will judge you and withhold His love from you. But He knows what you are dealing with before you do.

The lyrics in my song "Truth" speak to this:

> *I want to be honest with You, but I am so afraid,*
> *That if I tell You the truth, You might walk away.*
> *Should I just let things be and let You see what You must?*
> *But I'll be living a lie all because of pride.*
> *I'm stepping out on a limb, honesty starts within.*
> *So I'm going to tell You the truth.*

No matter what your weight in sin, why hide anymore? Why bear the burden alone? Why not be honest with the Lord? He already knows your pain and is waiting with outstretched arms to scoop you up and heal you.

That is, if you don't believe the lie. *You're beyond help,* whispers the enemy. *God won't get you out of this. Besides, you can handle it yourself.*

An unmarried former pastor told me a story that really helped me understand both the power of coming clean and the power of asking God for help.

His issue was lust.

The pastor had promised himself that he would acknowledge God in the midst of any temptation. He vowed that whenever he felt the urge to indulge his lust he would be honest with the Lord. He said, "Lord, whenever I'm in it, I'm going to admit that it's wrong."

One day he found himself alone with a beautiful woman he desired very much. Lust was overwhelming him. He wanted nothing more than to have sex with her. They were just a few zipper teeth away from the point of no return. And then he remembered his promise.

"Lord, I know what I'm about to do is wrong," he whispered aloud in the woman's ear. "But I'm going to go ahead . . ."

There's nothing like a confession of sin in your lover's ear to throw a wet blanket on a lust fest. After the words came out of his mouth, he and his almost-partner just stopped and looked at each other. Confessing the wrong stopped the wrong before it happened. Honesty stopped the sin cold.

But face it. Most of us aren't willing to be that honest. We take the easy way out and block the messages that don't support our decision to do whatever it is we are not supposed to do. We associate with people who support, abet, or condone our bad behavior. We filter out everything that doesn't align with our intention to do wrong. That's why the sound track for an adulterous relationship doesn't usually come from a Christian radio station. We choose *not* to fight the urge. We make a conscious decision to bar the Creator of the universe from the battlefield. We could say, "Lord, I want to pig out. I want a drink. I want to have sex with that person who isn't my spouse. Please take the urge from me." But we don't. We hide. And if we don't own the urge, the weight, the desire, the sin, we stay enslaved, insulated from the only power that can set us free.

## Blind Spots

I once heard a pastor say during a church service, "Whatever you don't handle now is going to show up in your destiny."

This applies to everyone: you, me, sports stars, entertainers, and presidents. Whatever weight in sin you're not dealing with now will keep trying to get your attention until you finally deal with it. Every time you ignore it, it comes back in a stronger and potentially more painful way. Ignore it for too long, and eventually, inevitably, it will show up as a personal catastrophe.

What was going to show up in my destiny? Would it be diabetes or a heart attack? Would I be gravely injured in a car wreck when I lost control of the vehicle while groping for a dropped french fry under the seat?

Stop hiding or die. I knew those were my options. I desperately wanted to be open to change so I could handle my destiny before it handled me.

Early in my weight-loss journey, I was attending an Italian church. There I was, a black guy trying to lose weight with a bunch of Italians. I was surrounded by mounds of food everywhere I turned.

A small group of us were studying Nehemiah. And then it occurred to me that my situation was not all that different from the one Nehemiah was in. Tired of seeing the land in ruins, he knew he had to do something. And as you know, that something was to mobilize a group to rebuild the wall to protect the once-glorious Jerusalem. In the process, he faced all kinds of obstacles.

One particular verse in chapter 4 really spoke to me:

*Meanwhile, our enemies were saying, "Before they know what's happening, we will swoop down on them and kill them and end their work."* —NEHEMIAH 4:11

When no one was looking, Nehemiah's enemies were going to attack where he least expected it. Then, says Nehemiah 4:12, the Jews who lived near the enemy overheard conversations and realized that Nehemiah's project was in real danger. They told

Nehemiah about what they'd heard. But they didn't just tell him once. They told him over and over. Some versions of the Bible say they told Nehemiah ten times. Then the lightbulb finally went on in Nehemiah's head, and he realized that he was vulnerable. So he fixed the problem. He put people with accountability into those exposed places to protect them. The project continued, and Nehemiah eventually finished the wall—in record time and under budget.

That got me thinking. Nehemiah had a blind spot. But the people who cared about him shouted and shouted until he could see his vulnerability and do something about it. I could imagine them yelling, "Hello! Wake up! This is important. I'm trying to tell you that the enemy is going to get you here! Not there, or there, but *here*. Where you least expect it."

The Jews were alerting Nehemiah to the fact that this was guerrilla warfare with a hidden enemy dedicated to derailing his project. The attacks would come from all the usual places, like ambitious politicians, but they would also come from unexpected places, like discouraged citizens and jealous secret rivals.

Like Nehemiah, I have blind spots. My weight was a big one, but it wasn't the only one.

Sometimes I wouldn't open credit card bills. I didn't know what I owed. I might owe the credit card company two thousand dollars, but when the statement arrived in my mailbox, I would think, *I just can't deal with this right now* and toss the unopened envelope in a drawer. Every statement was a shout from Nehemiah's friends. Every call from the collection agency was a shout from Nehemiah's friends. But it took more than ten times for me.

We all have blind spots that make us vulnerable to attack in exposed places. But instead of one hundred Jews shouting, "Wake up!" the voices are those of friends, mentors, the Holy

Spirit, and the Word. Other times the call to action doesn't come from people; it comes from the natural consequences of our secret weights in sin.

Your car just got repossessed. *Wake up!*

You gave your wife an STD. *Wake up!*

You gambled away the house payment. *Wake up!*

Your identity was stolen because you used your credit card to pay for online porn. *Wake up!*

You got fired because you stole from your employer. *Wake up!*

Nehemiah had to hear the message ten times before he woke up. I had to get to 475 pounds before I woke up. Some people never wake up. Some people never realize what they're carrying and how that load makes them vulnerable to attack.

The enemy takes advantage of our blind spots and uses them against us. *When you're not looking, I'm going to get you. I'm going to get you here. And here. And here.*

What will it take for you to wake up?

## Breaking the Silence

What will burst the bubble of denial and make you come clean? What will be the catastrophe that makes the scales fall from your eyes? What will make you go to the altar and confess your sins to the Lord so He can do what He has been waiting to do for you for so long? What will it take?

Is your blind spot keeping you from . . .

getting on the scale?

admitting the affair to your spouse?

confessing what you stole?

coming clean about drug or alcohol abuse?

showing your spouse the credit card bills?

Do you feel that you can't ask for God's help until you've solved the problem yourself? until you're perfect?

God wants you just as you are.

If you're overweight and saying, "I'll get it together first. I'll lose 15 pounds before I go in and weigh myself," you've got it backward. That's like wanting to get clean before you take a bath. It's like cleaning your house before the maid comes.

Your God is a loving God. He simply wants you to be honest. That message gets lost in some churches where everyone is obsessed with looking perfect and people are often afraid to be real.

I can remember one day when I was leading worship in church, and I just started singing out to the Lord, "Blow us away. Blow us away today. Do something different."

And boy, did He ever.

A young man went up and asked if he could speak. Pastor Steve gave him the microphone. And what he said astounded us all.

"I deal with an addiction to Internet pornography, and I hate it," he said, choking back the tears. "I don't want to do this anymore. I don't want it anymore."

A thousand people were in that service, but you could have heard a pin drop.

What happened next was amazing. Because this young man broke the silence, people began to flood the altar, confessing everything you can imagine. Until that man spoke and burst the bubble of shame, hundreds of people were sitting there, each crushed under his or her own weight in sin, each one feeling isolated, separate, and alone. But once the silence was broken, people couldn't wait to confess, and before long they were standing, kneeling, praying, and crying ten deep at the altar.

That worship service proved once again just how hungry we all are for God's healing—and how terrified we are to ask for it, especially in the presence of others.

It only takes one person speaking honestly to set into motion a chain reaction of healing. This young man had no fear of not looking perfect and no desire to censor himself to make it seem like everything was fine. He just got up there and spoke his truth in front of everyone: male, female, young, and old.

Nobody left the church that day thinking, *I'm so glad I'm not him.* No one left feeling superior. People left that church feeling lighter, cleansed, and less alone.

The pastor said very little that day. He just let the healing power of the Lord wash over the crowd. At the end of the service, he thanked me. "Calvin, I blame you for what happened here today," he said with a smile. "Because you asked the Lord to blow us away today, He did. And I thank you."

In my ministry, I have seen what happens when I share the unvarnished truth about my own struggles with weight. My honesty is a catalyst that gives others the courage to finally come to agreement with God that they are enslaved by destructive patterns of behavior.

The willingness to be honest—with yourself, with others, and with God—is all it takes for the healing to start.

What's stopping you from owning your weight in sin?

# CHAPTER 4

# STEP 2: SEE GOD AS YOUR FRIEND

PEOPLE ALWAYS TOLD ME how much God loved me. I just couldn't believe that it was true for me.

How could God love me? I messed up all the time—I was nowhere near perfect. I was a glutton. I lied. I stole. I cheated.

God might love other people—my good-hearted neighbor, my pastor, my mom—but there was no way He could love me.

I knew what was inside of me. I was so far away from the standard the Lord set for His people. I was too far gone. I was sure that God reserved His love for worthy people, those closer to perfection. Could God love me? No way. My mind was made up.

One day shortly after I had started my weight-loss journey, I was at a church service when the Lord whispered in my ear.

*Receive,* He said. *Just receive.* Later on, during prayer, I recalled one of my favorite verses:

*"I know the plans I have for you," says the* LORD. *"They are plans for good and not for disaster, to give you a future and a hope."*
—JEREMIAH 29:11

*Receive,* the Lord said again. *Don't you see? All you have to do is receive. I have a plan for your future, Calvin, and it's a good one.*

My first instinct was to argue. *No. It can't be true. You can't, because I'm not perfect.*

And then it hit me. I was arguing with the Creator of the universe.

God was telling me that He was going to make this wonderful promise come true for me if only I would receive it. But I wasn't willing to receive because I thought I knew better than the Lord. My beliefs about God were keeping me from receiving His wonderful promise for me. God kept knocking on the door, but I refused to let Him in because I refused to acknowledge that the door was even there. That's when the inspiration for my song "Receive" came to me.

> *Empty-handed I'm standing*
> *After striving so long.*
> *Unexpected I'm finding*
> *I don't have to be strong.*
> *Your grace is amazing,*
> *It's taken me so long*
> *To learn that Your love*
> *Has never been something I have to earn.*
> *Lord, I receive Your love*
> *Here in this moment.*
> *Your mercy flows like rain*
> *On my heart dry and broken.*

*I receive Your love today,*
*It's hard to believe that*
*All I must do is receive.*
*Sweet mystery,*
*All I must do is receive.*

## How Do You See God?

Is God a white-haired old man who looks like Charlton Heston? Is God your critical mother with the beehive hairdo in the food-stained muumuu? Is God your raging alcoholic father with bourbon-tinged breath raising his hand to smack you down and tell you that you're worthless? Is God an abusive babysitter who was supposed to care for you but didn't? Is God a trusted spiritual leader who betrayed you in the most intimate and irrevocable way? Is God someone in your life who keeps you from getting the things you deserve?

If you see God as a feared and despised authority figure, you are in good company. Authority figures from childhood loom larger than life in our memories, distorting the way we see people with power long after childhood ends. Maybe you had to tiptoe around your parents to keep the peace in the house. Maybe your teachers were abusive or neglectful. Maybe you tried to win their approval but couldn't.

When we view God through the lens of past relationships with authority figures, it's no wonder we're afraid to take our problems to Him. It's no wonder we view God less as a compassionate friend encouraging us to confide in Him and more like judge, jury, and executioner all rolled into one scary package up in the sky.

Who runs to a judge for comfort? No one I know. So instead

of rushing into the outstretched arms of our loving Creator, we sit in silence, shame, and embarrassment, certain that no one else is quite as bad, quite as irredeemable as we are, even though we hear people around us saying that they have finally accepted God's love for them. If you're like me, you might be thinking, *Yeah, that's all right for you, but it won't happen for me. God's love is for you, but not for me.*

Yes, we're embarrassed. Yes, we fear His disapproval. But the truth is, God cares about our pain. He cares about our hurts and our shame and our secrets. He cares about all this, and He is more than ready to love us when we come clean with Him.

## God Wasn't Born Yesterday

Nothing we tell God will surprise Him. The Lord has seen it all through the centuries.

The Bible is filled with examples of people who messed up. David made every mistake possible, it seems. He was a murderer, an adulterer, and a liar. He was broken. But the Lord loved David anyway because David brought his brokenness to Him.

I've always thought that David had a zipper problem. Even when he was on his deathbed, his handlers were bringing him virgins. Was he asking for them? Was that simply a perk of being the king? Was David just looking for comfort in all his usual ways, which meant acting out on a lifelong addiction to women? Was he being tempted to indulge his favorite comfort behavior until the very end?

I don't know what was going on with David, but I can tell you this: If I were on my deathbed and wanted to experience my favorite vice one last time, I wouldn't be asking for virgins. I would be asking for grits. Mounds of grits.

David had a lust issue, but he was still a man after God's own heart because he always came clean and asked for God's help. David trusted God with his secrets because he saw God as his comforter, not as his accuser.

The Bible holds the key to get you out of the but-not-for-me prison. Dig into God's Word and you'll find example after example of the Lord opening His arms to welcome back His wayward children. Is there judgment in the Bible? Yes, there's no getting around it. Wherever there is a hardened heart, there is judgment. But wherever hearts are softened with humility, acceptance, and repentance, God's loving hand is there, reaching out.

## Reliance or Defiance?

It's easy to conclude that we can manage this life just fine on our own. But in reality, every single thing that happens to us is designed to make us realize how much we need the Lord and to push us closer to Him.

Every interaction

Every triumph

Every tragedy

Every conversation

Every relationship

When I realized that God was allowing me to have both good and bad experiences in order to show me how much I really needed Him, it changed the way I looked at my weight in sin. Paul's experience recorded in 2 Corinthians 12:7-9 is a great illustration:

*To keep me from becoming proud, I was given a thorn in my flesh, a messenger from Satan to torment me and keep me from becoming proud. Three different times I begged the Lord to take it away. Each time he said, "My grace is all you need. My power works best in weakness."*

There are all sorts of theories about what Paul's thorn in the flesh might have been. Some scholars believe that he suffered from a medical condition such as epilepsy or migraines. Others believe he had trouble with his vision. Whatever it was, it was bad enough for Paul to ask God to remove it. In fact, he asked three times, and each time God refused.

What's my thorn? It is the way I cope with life. My default response to every challenge is to eat. Constantly dealing with that reminds me that I need God. Doing it my way got me to size 66.

The thorn is painful. I yank it out and give it to the Lord, only to realize that something else hurts. Now it's a tick buried in my arm, feasting on blood. Just after I've tweezed the little bugger out, I feel a sharp pain on the sole of my foot and realize there's a pebble in my shoe. I shake it out only to discover that I'm being stung by a wasp.

There's always a new challenge. God isn't a sadist. It's not that He doesn't love us. He allows us to have these experiences precisely *because* He loves us. He is testing us, refining us, and strengthening us. He gives us new challenges so we can have more opportunities to rely on Him.

Sometimes I think of God as the doctor who taps on your

knee with that little hammer during a physical exam. He's not hitting your knee to break you. He's not doing it because He wants to harm you. He's just testing your reflexes. And that six-inch needle that looks like a dagger? It isn't punishment for some wrongdoing; it's the delivery tool for a serum that will heal you.

The doctor is not out to kill us; He's here to help us. And that's how I view my relationship with the Lord. With my limited awareness, I can't always see that the situation, person, or thing that God has brought into my life will end up delivering the serum that will heal me.

## Perception Determines Reception

The way I perceive God determines the way I receive any communication from Him. I'm unlikely to believe or even welcome anything God says to me if I see Him as a judge.

It's easier for me to receive the truth from people when I know they love me. My friend Sal loves me unconditionally. My pastor loves me unconditionally. Because I know they love me and have my best interests at heart, I can accept their feedback.

If my pastor took me aside and said, "Calvin, you really need to look at yourself . . ." I would listen. It would hurt, but I would listen because I know he loves me and he is only trying to help me.

If I perceive that my pastor is spiritually grounded, then I receive his spiritual guidance. If I perceive that a friend is jealous of me, I am less likely to receive his comments.

When the leaders in my church in Pittsburgh "mentored" me about all my shortcomings, I had no desire to listen. *Wait a minute,* I thought. *You don't even know who I am. I just met you, and you're already rejecting me?*

God might have been trying to send me a message that day, but I didn't receive it because I believed the messengers were motivated by something other than love. They had bad news for me. It was news I needed to hear, but I was incapable of accepting it from people who had known me less than a week. Their bad news was wrapped in judgment.

A few years later I encountered another messenger from God who also had bad news. But this time the outcome was different. The messenger was my trainer, and the bad news was the reality of my weight. When my trainer weighed me the first time, he didn't make me feel like a bad or shameful person. He made me feel like he really understood. His bad news was wrapped in compassion, which said, *I love you unconditionally.*

It was God who motivated my trainer to help me avoid the humiliation of working out in a public gym. It was God who prompted him to rearrange his house so I could work out there.

> *Don't you see how wonderfully kind, tolerant, and patient God is with you? Does this mean nothing to you? Can't you see that his kindness is intended to turn you from your sin?*
> —ROMANS 2:4

My trainer delivered the change-course-or-die message with love and compassion. He went out of his way for me, which made me want to do right by him. I didn't want to disappoint him or make him think that his compassion was misplaced. I could see God working through my trainer—God with skin on. Finally, it really started to sink in how much God loved me and how lucky I was. And that understanding fueled my resolve to do better.

It's a lot like a husband whose behavior isn't the best in his marriage. He knows that his wife really loves him, but it just doesn't sink in. Maybe he has done things that aren't lovable. But when he realizes that she accepts his imperfections and extends forgiveness to him, he is so grateful that he wants to honor her and be the best person he can be. *This woman loves me,* he thinks, *even after all I've done to her.*

It's the same with God. After all we've done, He still loves us.

## Lies about God

Satan is a liar who wants us to believe that all this talk about God loving us is just a bunch of garbage. It's easy to forget that even if you have a personal relationship with Jesus Christ, the great deceiver is always out there doing his thing. If you're struggling with weight in sin, chances are good that you've forgotten that the enemy has one goal—to cut you off from God—and that he will do anything to accomplish that goal. The enemy is a master of subtlety, whispering something that sounds just enough like the truth to be believable. So you get sucked in to believing the lie that whatever God says isn't true. Here are my personal "favorites."

> **Lie #1: You are alone.** If you're like me and have a problem that everyone can see, your weight in sin is obvious. You only have to look around the mall to see that you're not alone. But the enemy is cunning. In my case, he worked overtime to make me believe that I was the only one on earth

whose eating was so out of control. He used my
friendships with normal-weight people to make
me feel like I was the only one with a problem.
He adjusted the filter settings in my brain so
I couldn't see the other overweight people who
were all around me. Recovery programs call
this "terminal uniqueness."

Lie #2: **There's something wrong with you.** The enemy
wanted me to believe that I was permanently
and totally flawed. *Other people might be fat,* the
enemy said, *but they're not fat for the same reason
you're fat. You're fat because there's something wrong
with you.* This lie is even more difficult to refute
if your weight in sin is hidden. No matter what
you are doing in secret—drinking, pornography,
heroin, bingeing, or shopping—the enemy wants
you to believe that you're the only one who has
ever done this, that you're worse than anyone else,
and that the people who love you would abandon
you if they knew the truth. *You aren't doing something wrong,* the enemy says. *You* are *wrong.*

Lie #3: **Nobody cares.** When I moved to Nashville
I didn't know anyone, but it didn't take long
for me to make friends. I knew that there were
people in this community who liked me. But
I still felt alone, especially on Sundays right
after church. In my hometown, Sundays had
always been a time for socializing and fun. But
in Nashville, most of my friends were parents

with young children, and their Sunday afternoon routines were different. When I invited friends to join me for an after-church meal, they would often say, "The kids have a game" or "The kids have to get a project ready for school." And they wouldn't invite me to join them, which was just the opening the enemy needed. *Man, nobody loves you. Nobody cares about you,* the enemy said. *If they did, you'd be at their house now.*

**Lie #4: You can't be all the way free.** *Real freedom from your weight in sin just isn't possible, so why try?* says the enemy, who wants us to believe that changing for the better means living a joyless, white-knuckle life of discipline and sacrifice. The enemy taunts us with thoughts of what we'll be missing if we give up our weight in sin. *Who wants to be that person who's always on a diet? Who wants to be that stick-in-the-mud who can't have any fun because he won't drink? Who wants to be that person who can't participate fully in all the pleasures life has to offer?* The enemy tells you that no one ever really recovers and that those who say they have are lying.

**Lie #5: Forgiveness? That's a bunch of baloney!** The enemy has a lot invested in keeping you far away from forgiveness, because he knows it is one of the most powerful tools in the spiritual toolbox. In fact, he works overtime to fill your head with all sorts of nonsense about what forgiveness is.

And he can be very convincing. *Forgiveness is just a word. It's resentment waiting to happen. Forgive, but don't forget. Forgiveness is for weak people—it's something you do when you're a door-mat. Forgiveness is something that other people get because—slap—remember, you're alone, you're too far gone, and nobody cares!* It's amazing to me how many believers accept without question that Christ died to secure their salvation but cling to the lie that the Lord won't forgive them for their weight in sin.

The enemy never stops lying, never stops trying, and never stops wooing. Every second of every day we get to choose whether we will believe the lie—or believe the Lord. What choice will you make?

## God Is for You, Not against You

It was December 31, 2000, and Pastor John, my former pastor in Cincinnati, was giving his New Year's Eve message.

The air was alive with the excitement of the watch night. A brand-new year with all its opportunity was on the horizon, but I was in another world. Doubt was in my mind. I was set to move to Nashville in five days, but was it the right thing to do? Was I moving for the wrong reasons? Was I just trying to run away from my problems in Pittsburgh?

I really felt that the Lord was calling me to make the move to Nashville, even though I had no idea what would happen to me there. At the same time, I could hear the voices of the elders in the church in Pittsburgh. I could remember every stinging criticism about my weight, not to mention the long list of other shortcomings they saw in me.

Was I doing the right thing?

Pastor John's booming voice jolted me out of my daze. "I've got three words for the New Year," he shouted. This was a man of God, a man of great spiritual power, and I respected him immensely. This was a man who heard from the Lord. What he said carried weight.

*Lord, please speak to me,* I prayed, desperately hoping that the pastor's words might hold some kind of answer. *I'm moving to Nashville in less than a week, and I really need to hear from You. And please shout.*

The excitement was building. Everyone around me was buzzing. *What are the three words? What are they?* The pastor was holding back, letting the sense of anticipation grow.

It was almost too much to bear. Just when I thought the crowd would erupt into a riot, the pastor yelled, "Okay, y'all, are you ready for these three words?"

All the people were on their feet jumping and shouting, "Yes! Yes! We're ready!"

The pastor paused for effect. "Now, I don't feel like this is really deep," he whispered into the microphone. "But I do feel like it is from the Lord." He paused again.

"Tell us!" someone screamed.

He smiled. "For the year 2001," he shouted, "the three words from the Lord are . . . Go. For. It."

The place went crazy! Around me, people were jumping up and down and hugging each other.

I had my answer. The Lord, working through this dramatic and charismatic pastor, was saying, *Do it. Go for it. I'm rooting for you!*

A few days later I moved to Nashville. And slowly but surely I went for it. The memories of that unforgettable watch night eventually found their way into a song called "God Is with You":

> *God is with you.*
> *God is for you.*
> *He is moving on your behalf.*
> *He is able to do much more*
> *Than you can ever think or ask.*
> *You don't have to be afraid.*
> *Know that He has made a way.*
> *For when your faith is extended,*
> *God will release His grace.*

## God's Will versus My Will

When I got to Nashville, I wanted a music career more than I had ever wanted anything. And I wanted it right away.

The Lord had other ideas. *Lose weight,* He said.

This wasn't what I wanted to hear. "What does my weight have to do with my voice?" I railed. "And while we're at it, Lord, I'm not all that happy down here. I'm not dating; I'm broke; I'm depressed. And You're telling me to lose weight? What else do You want from me?" Couldn't the Lord see that my career clock was ticking? I only had so much time to make something of my talent. If I didn't strike while the iron was hot, I would end up only singing at weddings on the weekends. Here I was, ready to launch my singing career, and the Lord was telling me to lose weight. I just didn't see the tie-in.

Little did I know that the Lord didn't want me to strike while the iron was *fat*!

I was chomping at the bit. "Lord, please make things happen for me," I prayed.

As usual, the Lord answered. *Trust Me; I have a strategy,* He responded. *Lose the weight first!*

I just didn't understand it. Music was what I really wanted to do, and I wanted to do it my way. Music first. Weight second. I looked at Luther Vandross. Barry White. They didn't have to lose weight to be successful.

But the Lord was persistent. *Look, I'm trying to bless you. I'm telling you to lose weight because I'm about to make all of this work for you. They're going to hear your music because of this. Trust Me.*

It didn't make any sense to me at the time. But instead of arguing that He was wrong or believing the lies, I shut up and listened. And now I can see. Had I tried to launch a music career without the weight loss, I wouldn't have gotten anywhere. It's not like I could have called Oprah and said, "Hey, sister, I'm a great singer, and I want to be on your show!" In reality, I was just another aspiring singer thinking he had something special.

God had other ideas. Actually, He had already written the business plan. Little did I know that I would eventually become more than just an aspiring singer. His plan for me would make me a messenger of hope, lighting the way for all who need to find a way out of their weight in sin, whatever that weight might be.

Who would have guessed that the Lord would ask me to lose weight first and then want me to talk to America about it, while taking my music with me? This wouldn't have been my plan! Who knew that He would use my journey from living under my own weight in sin and turn it around for His glory? Who would have dreamed that the Lord would use my act of surrender to help millions?

It just goes to show how little I know. Looking back, I'm grateful that I didn't insist on doing it my way. I'm glad I surrendered my weight in sin to the Lord, because I finally accepted the fact that God really does love me and He has a plan for me. All along, God cared about me and was intimately involved in my life. I just couldn't see it.

God cares about you, too. He wants to ease your pain. He cares about your hurts, your shame, and your secrets. His arms are open. Don't let your ideas about who He is keep you away.

CHAPTER **5**

# STEP 3: TAKE UP A NEW PERSPECTIVE

PEOPLE WHO ARE BURDENED by weight in sin often have trouble seeing the big picture. This is especially true for obese people.

When I first started my weight-loss program, I had no idea how I was going to get from where I was—200 pounds overweight—to where I wanted to be: a normal weight and a normal size. It just seemed like too far to go. It would take too long, and it would be too hard.

With a rush of enthusiasm, I had committed to giving my trainer ninety days. If I didn't lose the weight in ninety days, I would simply give up. But I didn't want to fail. I needed this to work. I was tired of playing diet games. I was sick of being huge, sick of hating myself, and sick of feeling stuck in life. I reasoned that if I couldn't stick it out for ninety days, I would resign myself to life as a super obese person and die a slow death.

Would it work? Could I do it? I had never been serious about losing weight before. But there I was, committing nights, weekends, and holidays from January to April. I didn't have to think about May or June or next year; I simply had to worry about getting through the day and stringing ninety of them together.

My trainer took a picture of me on the first day of our work together, the "before" shot that would serve as a visual benchmark of my progress. It was terrifying to see the evidence of how bad things really were, but I had faith in my trainer and in the process.

*Ninety or nothing. Ninety or nothing,* I kept telling myself. Every day I looked at myself in the mirror, and every day I saw the same thing. Fat Calvin. Rock head. After nearly a month, I began to get discouraged. Where was the transformation? I was working out, eating right, and making small changes in my lifestyle and habits. And I was seeing nothing in the way of change. How was I going to keep this up if nothing improved?

"Keep going," said my trainer, gently urging me to focus on other things. "You promised me ninety days, and you haven't even hit thirty. You have more than sixty to go."

On day thirty, my trainer had a surprise for me. "Get ready for your close-up," he said. He took another picture and compared it to the one we had taken on the first day.

"Look," he said. "Can you see the difference?"

I couldn't see the difference at all. I was too big to be weighed on the scale, and I was still wearing my size 60 jeans. However, I was determined to honor my commitment to the ninety-day process.

Near day ninety, I went to my friend Sharon's wedding. Many of our mutual friends hadn't seen me in a while, and they were all over me. "There's something different about you," said one friend, looking me up and down. "What's happening? Did you shave your mustache? Did you cut your hair? Wait! Have you been losing weight?"

After the third person approached me like that, I knew it was really happening. It was working. The success strengthened my commitment. Broken down into ninety-day increments, the journey didn't look that bad. Instead of obsessing about getting from here to minus 200, I could just focus on getting from January to April.

At the ninety-day mark, I started to see how the Lord was going to connect the dots for me. I was finally starting to see the big picture and God's vision for my life. I felt like I had climbed a mountain and was now able to see where I was in relation to where I wanted to be. It looked like a really long journey, but I knew I didn't have to do it all in one day. I had committed to starting somewhere, and I had piled one day on top of the next and one ninety-day period on top of another. I knew it would eventually all add up to big change.

As for the master plan, that was no longer my concern. I had stopped trying to run the show. My own best efforts had gotten me to somewhere just south of 500 pounds. My job was to suit up, show up, grow up, and leave the driving to God.

Now that I could see where I was going, I had to admit that the view was mighty fine. I was going to be thin. I was going to turn my misery into a ministry of hope, and I would blend my story and song into a powerful catalyst for change. Oprah would invite me to be on her show, where I would tell my story and sing my songs. I would perform on all kinds of programs. I would be a household name, and it would all be for God's glory.

All of a sudden my weight in sin started to look like a blessing rather than a curse. When I started to see God's vision for me—that He was planning to use me as an instrument to spread the word about Him—all my misery started making sense, and God's vision became my vision. I now had a purpose.

## The Power of Purpose

I have always been a person who needed a reason to do something. I have always wanted to know why. Once the *why* of my misery—God's purpose for me—became apparent, it was exciting. I was passionate about reaching the goal, which made me focus on doing everything I could to be successful. Knowing the purpose set in motion a chain reaction of excitement and focus that made me unstoppable.

I once heard Pastor James Ryle summarize that kind of chain reaction in this way: "Vision breeds passion, and passion breeds discipline."

Let's take an example many of us can relate to. A woman is getting married on October 5. It's July 28, but she knows she has a dress to fit into. She's passionate about her wedding, and she's making all the right eating choices wherever she goes because she bought that dress in the size she is *going* to be.

That kind of vision kept me going. I was passionate about it, which made me disciplined. When someone asked me, "Hey, do you want some cake?" the answer was no. And it felt so good! I could see how this simple act of saying no fit into my larger plan, even when the cake was offered by the generous and loving Italians in my home church. I could see how saying no to that cake was like a cog in the wheel that was gaining momentum by the day. I was on a roll, and I didn't want to go back.

It's easy to make the right food choices when you have a vision. And the resulting success seeps into every part of life. Dr. Myles Munroe, founder, president, and senior pastor of Bahamas Faith Ministries International, puts it this way: "Where purpose is not known, abuse is inevitable." He tells a story to prove his point.

A couple owned a stately old home in a tree-lined part of town. A beautiful tree in the front lawn gave the house its unique curb appeal. But one day, to their horror, the home owners discovered that their home was infested with termites. They called an exterminator to inspect the damage.

"You have two options," he said after surveying the couple's property. "Either get rid of that tree or bring in cockroaches."

The home owners looked at each other and then at the exterminator. Cockroaches?

"That's right," said the exterminator. "The presence of the cockroaches cancels out the presence of the termites. The tree or the termites: the choice is yours."

I don't remember what the home owners in the story ended up doing, but Dr. Munroe made his point loud and clear. Most of us believe that cockroaches don't have a purpose. They don't make sense to us. They're dirty, they're a nuisance, and we don't like them. In fact, we try to kill them.

But everything in God's creation has a purpose, even cockroaches. Since we don't understand the purpose of a cockroach, abuse is inevitable. The roach motel comes to mind.

Think about your own life. Think about the people you encounter and the situations you find yourself in. If you don't know their purpose, abuse is inevitable.

I once heard Dr. Munroe cite another example of this principle. "What happens when you give a two-year-old a Rolex watch?" he asked. "A two-year-old doesn't know the purpose of a Rolex, so he's going to abuse it. He's going to step on it and use it as a hammer and drool on it."

The same could be said about your day-to-day life.

You could be eating dinner at a nice restaurant after a very, very bad day at work. You take out your frustrations on your server. You don't mean to do it, but there you are, yelling at her and acting like a jerk. But what if you found out that she was really a gifted entertainer who is just a few weeks from her big break? You'd probably treat her differently, right? Everyone deserves to be treated well, because everyone has a specific purpose.

This new way of looking at people, places, and things changed my life. It altered my perspective and taught me the importance of not overlooking people. It showed me that I need to pause and consider what their purpose might be. Where might they be going? Who might they become?

This applies to you, too, not just to others. If you don't know the purpose for your life—and vision is purpose, in my book— then abuse is inevitable. The people, places, and things in your life just won't make sense.

And when you don't understand the purpose of your life, there is a good chance that you will abuse yourself in the ways you have come to see as comfort: food, sex, drugs, alcohol, relationships, spending, and more.

As the weight fell off, I started to see that my problem all along was a problem of vision. I think it's the same for many of us. We don't know what God's vision for us really is, so we feel like we have no purpose. And if there's no purpose, why not live for the moment? Why not satisfy every selfish desire, act on every crazy whim? Why not have that binge, act on that lustful urge, spend money we don't have, or finish that fifth of whiskey? Why not do what feels good? It's easy to just give up when we don't have vision.

What is your purpose? What is your reason for living a better life?

## Get a New Perspective

When you combine a vision for your future with a new perspective, your life will change dramatically.

Mine did.

What is perspective? Perspective is your point of view. It's the way you see things, and this makes all the difference when it comes to living life without your old familiar friend: your weight in sin.

Let's look at an example. Mel Gibson's stunning film *The Passion of the Christ* is a great study in perspective. Had Gibson chosen to tell his tale from only one point of view—say, the mother's—the result could have been a forgettable movie about a mom who loses her son.

But Gibson's tale unfolds from three perspectives: the enemy's, the disciples', *and* the mother's. The result is a story far richer, far more compelling, and far more instructive than it would have been if it had been told from a single point of view.

The way you see a situation might seem like the only way to look at it. But it isn't. There is more than one way to look at reality, and it's not necessarily the way you are looking at it.

Here's another example. Take this book—my book—that you're reading right now. From where you're sitting, you can see the words. But a person watching you read the book will see something else. If you're reading a hard copy of this book, the person sitting across from you will see the cover. If you're reading this book on a computer, he will see the back of your laptop or PDA. Either way, that person won't see the contents. He won't see the message. Let's say this person gets frustrated because he can't see the contents. What would you tell him to do? You might ask him to join you and look at the book for himself. And then, suddenly, he would be able to see what he couldn't see before. Simply because he got up and moved.

That's a change in perspective. It's moving from where you are to a different place so you can see something in a new way.

Changing your perspective takes practice. But the first step is admitting that your view of a situation might not be the only way to look at it. Sometimes I find it helpful to imagine myself stepping out of my body and looking at an issue from a different place. Other times I will actually stop thinking about the problem, stand up, and go somewhere else before I start thinking about the situation again. Often a physical change of scenery or a short break from thinking about the problem is all it takes to help me look at a problem in a new way.

To change my perspective, I do other things as well.

*I talk to others.* Telling someone I trust about my situation and asking that person for feedback is a great way to get another viewpoint. Because the other person is not me, his or her perspective is automatically going to be different. At times I am astounded by what I hear when I have the courage to share my problems with others.

*I dig into God's Word.* Count on the Bible for the right perspective every time, no matter what the situation. If I'm having trouble dealing with a weight in sin, I go to my concordance and look up all the verses that relate to my situation. I then read them all. Some fit my situation and some don't. But no matter what, somebody in that book has been through what I'm going through, and the answer will be there.

*I talk to and listen to God.* There's nothing like a personal relationship with the Lord to give you a new perspective. Time in prayer—thanking Him for all He has done so far, sharing my feelings about the situation, laying the situation at His feet, expressing gratitude in advance for the way He will work in this situation, and listening for His guidance—is absolutely essential.

## Life through God's Eyes

New perspectives don't come to a closed mind. Spiritual insights don't occur in hardened hearts. If I'm certain that there's just one way to view a problem in my life, I am not open to alternative viewpoints. And if I'm not open to alternative viewpoints, that means I'm also not open to God's viewpoint. Being who He is, the Lord honors my request and lets me continue doing things my way, blind to the new information His perspective might give me—even if it's the very information I need to solve the problem.

God wants us to look at everything differently, even the pain caused by facing our weight in sin. He wants us to see ourselves the way He sees us. And He is willing to help us do this if we don't let our stubborn pride get in the way.

My song "Bigger" speaks to this.

> If it's bigger than me then it must be You,
> Because all of my strength, Lord, it just won't do.
> There's a lesson to learn while I'm going through,
> 'Cause I want to see things the way You do.
> Above the clouds the sun is still shining,
> The rain will pass and I'll shine, too.

These lyrics came to me during a flight. I was returning to Nashville, and we were just starting our final descent. We were high above the clouds, which were exploding into vertical puffs that looked like a giant cotton ball convention in the sky. It was beautiful, though it was hard to keep looking out the window because the sun was so bright.

We continued to descend, and the plane sank into the clouds. Dark gloom replaced the brilliant sunshine. Just like that. It was so dark it looked like it would rain, and then suddenly we were through the clouds and back in the sun again. When we were on the ground, I thought, *Wait a minute. What I see might not be reality . . . at least not for long.*

Sometimes the only thing needed to change our perspective is time. A simple landing showed me that. The only thing that changed was the airplane's position. The outlook seemed gloomy for only a few minutes, and when we moved through it, I could see the reality that had always been there—the sun just beyond the clouds.

I'm one of those people who let the weather affect my mood. When it's dreary, I can get depressed. I think it's going to be blah forever, and I forget that the sun will come out again.

Reality isn't always what we think it is. We don't see things the way they are; we see them the way *we* are. Reality is always there—just beyond our limited perspective—waiting for us to discover it. And our Lord is eager to help.

Taking on a new perspective meant choosing to see the *real* reality. The sun was out. It was just on the other side of the clouds. Soon the clouds would part and the sun would return.

## Reframing the Past

Taking on a new perspective is especially valuable if you struggle with things that happened in the past. Yes, the past is done. It's over with. You can't change a thing that happened. But you aren't completely powerless over the past. You can change the way you look at it.

Has something really bad happened to you in the past? Have you had a personal tragedy occur that you just can't forget?

Maybe you feel bad about the way you were raised. Maybe your parents did the best they could, but—let's face it—in spite of their best efforts, you still felt overly sensitive and insecure. All the slings and arrows of life that seemed to bounce off others ended up hurting you. Maybe the pain was so great that you ended up needing doughnuts and grits to shield yourself against the disappointment, the rejection, and the discouragement.

Maybe you wonder if your parents are in some way responsible for the fact that you turned out this way. Maybe on some level you blame them. After all, if they had encouraged you more, gone to your ball games, stuck up for you more, supported your interests, bought you better clothes, lived in a bigger house, driven a nicer car, and been cool like the other parents, maybe you wouldn't have this terrible weight problem. If they had spent more time and energy showing you what was possible instead of focusing so much on what you couldn't do, maybe life would be better.

If only your upbringing had been different, maybe you wouldn't feel quite so enslaved by appetites you can't control. Maybe you wouldn't spend so much time and energy always trying to get more—more food, more things, more approval, more whatever—to make life less painful.

Okay, you've probably figured it out by now. This is me I'm talking about.

Can you see how easy it is to get stuck?

*If only things had been different.* I sigh, feeling the wave of self-pity wash over me.

Hello! From where I sit today, there isn't a thing I can do about my past. But I can change the way I view it. I can change my perspective. If you are like most people—like me—you will have trouble doing this on your own. You will need supernatural help, the kind only the Lord can offer. Talking to trusted advisers, spending time in solitude with the Word, and talking with God in prayer are good ways to start the process. But there's more you can do. There's one essential ingredient that can't be overlooked: gratitude.

God commands us to be thankful for everything. Here is how I do it.

**I am grateful for what I've been given.** God tells us to be grateful for everything, but sometimes it's hard to be grateful for things that seem bad. The truth is, however, that those situations were placed in our paths to make us who we are today. My parents gave me many things that I am very grateful for—things like a big heart, a generous nature, and musical ability. I can choose to dwell on the things I'm lacking, or I can focus on the things I've been given.

**I am grateful for what I have *not* been given.** With my virtually nonexistent boundaries and people-pleasing tendencies, I used my weight to protect me from all sorts of evils. I could have gotten into drugs or fornication or worse. I think every day about the trouble I could have gotten into—and I got into plenty even with my weight as a shield—and I am grateful for God's protection. I am even grateful for the fact that I didn't have much in the way of self-esteem. That's the reason I didn't start singing until college, and I think that God was protecting me. If I had started singing earlier without the weight-loss story to tell, my identity might have been wrapped up in my music instead of in my ministry. I might have been healthier, but I would have been a different person.

**I am grateful for what was taken away.** God removes things when we're ready and not a second earlier. When I realized that God was going to use my weight-loss story for His glory, I was able to see one of the reasons I had been given the burden in the first place. And then, as my surrender grew, the weight fell off. Rejection is God's protection, and it took me many years to see how true that was.

Changing my perspective on the past healed my relationship with my parents. Today I can see that they did the best that they could. It wasn't that they didn't want to give me what I needed; they simply didn't know how. We are all just making it up as we go along. Even our parents. Now they're my biggest fans, and I love them.

Changing my perspective meant reframing my past and looking at it as a source of strength rather than a burden to overcome. When you get right down to it, I am the way I am because of the pain I've gone through. If I had to do it all over again, I wouldn't change anything.

Today I am grateful for every hardship, challenge, and disappointment I have gone through, because the pain these difficulties created is the very thing that enables me to connect with people on such a deep level. My pain is the source of the gift I give to others, and it's the reason people open up to me. Ultimately, it's the conduit God uses to reach people who so desperately need His love, grace, and mercy.

A new perspective helps me realize that without the struggle, there would be no story. It can be the same for you.

# CHAPTER 6

# STEP 4: GET SOMEONE TO HOLD YOU ACCOUNTABLE

THE BIGGER YOUR WEIGHT IN SIN, the harder it is to stay motivated and keep handing the problem over to God. My weight in sin was mammoth size. I had 200 pounds to lose. I knew that it would be hard to stay motivated for a few days, let alone the months and years needed to lose all the weight. I needed help staying focused.

And that's why when I decided to hire a personal trainer, I thought of Jeff. We worked together as worship pastors, and Jeff's demeanor was both disarming and appealing. Women often referred to him as a hunk, and rightly so. Jeff looked like Sylvester Stallone before the *Rocky* franchise entered its geriatric phase. But he defied the bodybuilder stereotype. He didn't seem vain or self-obsessed.

This wasn't the first time I approached Jeff about my situation. About a year before I made the commitment to pick up change, I had learned that he did some personal training on the side. Would he be willing to help me? I was almost afraid to ask.

One day I mustered the courage. "I'm a little out of shape," I admitted, praying he wouldn't burst out laughing at the understatement. "Will you work with me?"

He said he would, but it ended before we really even got started. He put me on a food plan that involved drinking tasteless shakes. I hated it. It wasn't working, so I gave up. Jeff was gracious about it and just let me go without any negative judgment.

Now I realized that my failure didn't have anything to do with those horrible shakes. It was me. It wasn't that the food plan didn't work; it was me who didn't do the work. I hadn't been ready to give up my best friend, my comforter, my counselor, my wonderful. I wasn't ready to give up the food.

But that wasn't all. I was also afraid of being held accountable. I didn't want to make a promise to myself—or worse yet, another person—and then have to admit that I had broken it. I didn't want to lose weight and then worry about people snickering behind my back when I started gaining again. I wanted the freedom to blow my diet and not have anyone call me on it. I wanted to be exempt from the consequences of my actions. *The laws of physics that govern the conversion of food to energy shouldn't apply to me,* I thought. I should be one of those people who can eat whatever they want and never gain weight. I didn't want to have to report to anyone like a child. I didn't want to have to be honest about how much I was eating and how little I was moving. And most of all, I didn't want anyone telling me what to do. *You are not the boss of me!* That was my credo.

I'm certain that Jeff could see right through me. He had heard all the excuses. And as an ordained minister, he had sharp spiritual acuity. Personal trainers and spiritual leaders meet people every day who claim to want results, as long as it doesn't involve change, honesty, or effort.

This had always been my problem. I didn't really want to change, I wasn't willing to be honest (especially with myself), and I was unwilling to put forth effort for very long. In the past, I had always run from any situation where I might be held accountable—at work, in relationships, and with my weight. But when I was finally ready to pick up change, I prayed that this time things would be different.

## Why Use a Trainer?

I have always been complacent. *What's the least I can do to get by? That's what I'll do.* This approach may work for some things in life, but when you have 200 pounds to lose, the bare minimum simply won't cut it. That's when a trainer becomes really valuable.

> **A trainer pushes you to do more.** My natural tendency is to look for the shortcut. Trainers have pushed me outside of my comfort zone physically, emotionally, and mentally over the years. Many times they encouraged me to keep going when I wanted to quit. Not long ago, I was working out with my pastor, Steve. We were in the middle of a workout that involved running down a hallway, picking up a cone, and bringing it back. We had to do this three times. But when it was my turn, I walked down the hallway, picked up all three cones, and brought them closer so I wouldn't have to go so far the next two times. The trainer saw me. "Oh! Calvin is cheating!" he said. We laughed about it, but he was right. There is a part of me that is always looking for an exit. A trainer blocks the exit and keeps you going.

A trainer teaches you new things. I thought I knew how to eat right, but I didn't. I thought I knew what kind of exercise was right for me, but I didn't. I thought I knew what my limits were, but I didn't. If you are teachable—willing to let go of all your old ideas—you will learn a lot from your trainer. A good trainer will advise you on two of the most important aspects of physical care: what you put in your mouth and how you move your body. If you're willing to follow instructions, you will learn things you can use for the rest of your life. Things like:

- Vegetables taste great when they're prepared in certain ways.
- Healthy food can fill you up.
- Exercise won't kill you.

I don't really know what it was that made me think that learning new things would be so difficult. I was convinced that it would be a bad experience. But because my trainer broke the new concepts down into bite-size pieces and fed them to me without judgment, I was able to take the new information and use it.

**A trainer motivates you to keep going.** When I first started to work out with Jeff, I wanted to quit all the time. But I didn't want him to think I couldn't do it. At times I felt like I was working out as much for him as for me because I respected and admired him so much. I didn't want to disappoint him. On some days that was the only thing that kept me going. And after I had lost about 125 pounds, when I started to feel complacent, he pushed me to keep going. He motivated me without bullying me. He simply encouraged me to honor the promise I had made to myself. Eventually I, too, believed that I could go all the way.

**A trainer encourages you.** Obese people can be very fragile. Encouragement that sounds even the least bit like bullying, rejection, or disrespect can be very destructive. Jeff knew that, and his ability to keep me focused on what I could do was empowering. It made me want to change. His gentle encouragement was a model for me, and his approach is the one I use today. When I say, "You can do it!" to a struggling person, it's Jeff's voice I'm imitating, as he said those same words to me. Jeff was able to walk the tightrope between encouragement and accountability with finesse. Somehow he was able to be stern yet gracious at the same time.

## Put Your Money Where Your Mouth Is

The people Jeff trained for free rarely stuck with it. Only those who were willing to make an investment remained truly committed. That's why I didn't want him to train me for free. I knew that if I didn't put some skin in the game, so to speak, I wouldn't do the work.

*Wherever your treasure is, there the desires of your heart will also be.* —MATTHEW 6:21

Hiring a trainer was a big sacrifice for me. How would I pay for it? I didn't have any extra money. And then I realized that I always seemed to have plenty of money when I:

- placed my order at the fast food drive-up window
- picked up the check in my favorite restaurants
- stood in the checkout line to buy boxes, bags, and bins of binge foods

I could always find money to feed my addiction. That's when it occurred to me that I could afford to do anything I wanted to do if I made that thing a priority. I *could* afford a trainer if I made changing my life a higher priority than getting my food fix. I had a lot more money than I realized when I factored in what I was spending on food. For me, paying for my personal training, and making it a priority, was just another way of holding myself accountable.

## Getting the Most from Your Trainer

How can you make your investment pay off to the greatest extent? Here are a few tips that come directly from my personal experience.

**Make a commitment.** Work with your trainer to choose a defined period for your training. Give it an end date. Mine was ninety days. If there's an end point, you have a finish line. At that time, you can decide if you want to keep going. String those short-term commitments together, and you have big change.

Take the long view. Jeff told me that we were going to sow seeds into my life and that I would reap a lifestyle as a result. This wasn't a diet, he said—this was a way of living. You go on a diet and then you go off. Without wholesale changes in my lifestyle, I would go off the diet the second I fit into my test pants, and then my weight would begin to climb again.

**Get structure.** Shortly after starting to work with Jeff, I took a temporary job at an investment company. It was one of the best things I could have done. As a creative person, I don't have much discipline. Off-the-cuff living is what I do best, especially when I am working on my music. But being in the corporate world was exactly what I needed in the early part of my training. It gave my days a new kind of structure. Jeff wanted me to exercise before work, so I had to get up earlier to walk on the treadmill. I knew that I would eat lunch at a certain time and that I could get my meals cooked to order at the company's on-site cafeteria. I—off-the-cuff Calvin—actually had a routine.

**Surrender to discipline.** I have trouble following orders. I really hate it when people tell me what to do. But the truth is that my resistance to discipline is nothing more than rebellion. Without owning up to that simple truth, I wouldn't have been able to follow my trainer's directions. But if I rebel whenever someone tries to tell me what to do, then I'm stuck. I'm unteachable and closed to new ideas, which means nothing can change. I had to stop looking for the line and trying to cross it. Fortunately, though he was sensitive and loving, Jeff wasn't a softy. He didn't let me get away with anything.

**Expect discomfort.** I really didn't want to have to push myself too hard, especially physically. So when my trainer asked me to begin by walking just fifteen minutes every other day, I balked. My parents had even purchased a treadmill for me, but I still resisted. Fifteen minutes every other day? It was just too much! Because I was so big, I sweated easily. Sweat would drip down my face, stain my shirt, and dribble down my back. Jeff knew that I didn't like discomfort, but he pushed me to lean into it instead of running away from it. He often called me at 5:30 a.m. and said, "C'mon, Calvin. Get up! Walk!" When I started strength training, my body wasn't used to the effort and I experienced a lot of discomfort. I felt like I was going to throw up. But I kept going. I also experienced emotional discomfort. The thought of working out in front of other people was mortifying, so I worked out at Jeff's house. The prospect of facing life without all my favorite foods was difficult. When you're an emotional eater, putting down your drug means facing life on life's terms. And that's where I found that I really need God.

## Fear of Success

As the weight began to come off, I wrote to the company whose supplements I was using and told them about my success. Representatives from the company contacted me and asked if they could use my testimony and pictures in an ad campaign. At first I was excited, but then I started to worry. If my picture and story were splashed across billboards and magazines, what would happen if I gained the weight back? The more I made it obvious that I was losing weight, the more I risked being ridiculed if I failed. After all, a lot of people find smug satisfaction when someone's weight-loss attempts fail. I know the enemy does.

The company representative tried to soothe my fears. "Why don't you want to help people?" he asked. "Your experience could inspire millions to change their lives for the better. Are you afraid of success?"

The more I thought about it, the more I realized that those pictures would make me accountable in a very public way. If I gained the weight back, everyone would know. So yes, the company rep was right. I was afraid of success, but most of all I was afraid of being held accountable.

This fear continued to be an obstacle. I resisted the idea of building a ministry around my experience. For years I knew that I would need to tell my story. But how could I do it without having to be accountable? *Please, God,* I prayed, *I know You want me to tell my story, but please don't make me go public with this. Don't make me put myself out there only to face embarrassment and rejection if I get fat again.*

But God had other ideas. And He has a sense of humor. *Calvin,* He said to me one day while I was praying, *this thing you're really afraid of—being accountable in a really public way—is the very thing I'm going to use to help you keep the weight off. I'm going to make your fears and your pride work for you, not against you.*

I should have seen it coming. Ministry out of misery. Lemonade out of lemons. That's what the Lord does.

## Finding the Right Trainer

So what should you look for in a trainer? Here's what I have learned:

**A good trainer must have credibility.** Jeff had it; another trainer I worked with didn't. Jeff walked the talk; my other trainer didn't. The other trainer didn't hold me accountable for what I ate, and he allowed foods that were clearly binge triggers for me. *You're just giving me more freedom because you don't want to hold yourself accountable,* I thought after observing how he worked out and what he ate. It was the old "Do as I say, not as I do."

**A good trainer must be certified.** Has this person worked with others with similar challenges, abilities, and limitations to yours? If your weight is starting in the high numbers, as mine was, it's even more important that your trainer have the skills, experience, and education necessary to train you safely.

**A good trainer should be spiritually aware.** Notice that this is a "should" rather than a "must." As an ordained minister, Jeff brought a spiritual dimension to the training experience. It was Jeff's influence that really helped me make the connection between my physical weight and the weight in sin between my ears. Most of our burdens have a spiritual component. In fact, most addictions are simply attempts to fill that God-shaped hole in our souls. When your trainer can link the spiritual with the physical, it rockets your recovery into a new dimension.

**A good trainer is compassionate.** Tough love only goes so far with obese people. If you have a lot of weight to lose, the ideal trainer is compassionate, encouraging, and gentle—but also doesn't let you whine, at least not for long. It's a fine line. Personal problems might make you want to blow your diet, skip training sessions, or complain constantly. A good trainer will listen to your concerns, gently offer suggestions, and get your focus back on your training.

## The Power of the Village

My trainer wasn't the only person I relied on. It took a network of accountability partners to keep me on the straight and narrow. No matter what your weight in sin, the same will be true for you. Accountability was the key that unlocked the door for me to walk away from desperation and into freedom.

The song "Mercy Is on Its Way" speaks to this. I wrote this song for an organization called Mercy Ships, which sends non-government hospital ships to third world countries. Doctors on board heal people through surgical procedures that aren't accessible locally.

When I first learned about Mercy Ships, I cried. I thought about my own journey and how the people in my life—my trainer, my family, and my friends—had been like a Mercy Ship to me. Without them, I might be dead now.

The lyrics for "Mercy Is on Its Way" come from my own pain, but they could just as easily apply to the pain of a person in a third world country who desperately needs physical healing and can't get it. They can also apply to the pain of anyone struggling with a burden he or she can't seem to shake.

> *I was lost in desperation, crying out for some relief,*
> *Wondering in times of silence,*
> *Would this be the end of me?*
> *Heaven send someone to help me,*
> *Erase the past and now I'm free.*

*Love has found me here, heard my every prayer,*
*Hope knows my name,*
*Everything changes today, mercy is on its way.*

The Lord sent people to help me. My closest friends still serve as my accountability partners. I call them my Sin Management Squad. They keep me honest, and I really need them. My capacity for self-delusion is bottomless, and my friends see right through my denial at times when I can't or won't.

These are people who love me unconditionally. I'm not afraid to be vulnerable with them and let them see the truth about my life behind the facade. They aren't afraid to tell me bad news or prop me up if necessary to keep me on the right path.

When I tell my friend Sal that I'm having trouble making healthy food choices while on the road, he doesn't give me food tips. "How's your prayer life?" he asks me. "Are you reading the Word?"

Sal knows that if I'm spiritually fit, my desire to take back my weight in sin will diminish. He, like all my accountability partners, shines the bright light of the Spirit in the dark corners of my heart, exposing the blind spots that threaten to keep me enslaved.

And Sal doesn't stop there. When I'm on the road, he sends me text-message reminders about what passages I should be reading. Instead of getting irritated because Sal is telling me what to do, I just follow instructions. It's so much easier that way.

Even when you have good accountability mechanisms in place and you have spiritual momentum, it's easy to become complacent. It's easy to look at others and feel superior. It comes on gradually, sometimes so gradually that I don't even realize it. *So many people love my music. I know more of the Bible than they do, so I don't need to read it every day.*

But it only takes one look from one of my accountability partners to bring me back to reality, especially if I'm talking to them about my struggles with food choices or my resistance to working out. "Calvin," they say, "don't believe your own PR. Here you are, dying because you can't stop eating, and you think you don't need to get into God's Word? Wake up!"

Sometimes it takes a two-by-four to the head to wake me up.

No matter what your weight in sin, the process works the same way. Simply

admit the weakness and how it is devastating your life

surrender the weakness to the Lord

find accountability partners

be honest with them at all times

I've tried to follow this process in my own life. I've listed my weaknesses, just to be honest with myself. And then I have found people to help me be accountable in those areas. I actually have different people I rely on for support in different areas. My pastor holds me accountable spiritually, but I look to a mentor for help with my creative issues. When you're living in the Lord's will for you, your life will be rich and varied, which means you will need a lot of loving people around you to be your advisers. It takes a village.

## Give It Away in Order to Keep It

My accountability partners remind me that to whom much is given, much is required. Today my work as a speaker, an author, and a singer gives me plenty of opportunities to give back. Most satisfying is the work I do one-on-one with people who are suffering. I also like to sit down with their friends and family to show them how to help their loved ones with their struggles.

I once helped a seventeen-year-old boy lose 100 pounds. Though the work was his to do, it was his family—the people around him—who held him accountable. His parents, siblings, aunts, and uncles stayed by his side, stocked the house with healthy foods, kept him honest, and kept him focused on the goal. It's this spirit of community that makes accountability such a powerful thing. It gives us direct access to the Creator of the universe, who empowers us to thumb our noses at the enemy when he whispers, *You're all alone in this. . . . No one is looking, so why not just have that half gallon of ice cream? C'mon, you deserve it.*

The bottom line is that no matter what our weight in sin, God provides people along the path to encourage us, challenge us, and most important, keep us accountable. We don't have to do it alone.

# CHAPTER 7

# STEP 5: START SOMEWHERE

1. Promise to change.
2. Try to change all at once.
3. Get discouraged and fail.
4. Give up.
5. Rinse and repeat.

If I were a bottle of shampoo, these would be the instructions. This was the way I lived my life, and not just with my weight. I got stuck in the same self-defeating thought patterns when I was starting my music career. Here's an example:

**Me:** I have a dream. When I record my CD, I will be slim, because there's no way I'm going to be fat on the cover. I'm starting my diet in the morning.

**Enemy:** That's a great idea. I'm right here with you.

**Me:** I can do it! I know I can. I'm going to eat right and exercise and be good. Starting tomorrow, I'm going to walk two miles a day and eat less.

**Enemy:** You'll lose faster if you commit to five miles a day and don't eat anything until dinner.

**Me (pausing to think):** Okay. If a little is good, more is better, right?

**Enemy:** Sure. Why not start big? Hasn't it been a while since you ate? It's dinnertime. How about a snack to tide you over?

**Me:** Uh, okay. Just one.

**Enemy:** Now that you've had one, you might as well eat the whole thing. After all, you've messed up *again*!

**Me:** (chewing sounds, bag rustling)

If I had a penny for every time that dialogue happened in my head, I could pay off my car.

The enemy kept me from taking that first tiny step with my weight by convincing me that I had to do it all at once. He tried to tell me that the only way to reach the goal was to make gigantic changes. Deep down I knew that it was possible to change, but I couldn't see any way to get there. Because the enemy would encourage me to set impossible goals, I always tried and then quickly failed. Eventually I just stopped trying.

I had so much weight to lose that it seemed impossible for me to stick with it long enough to even make a dent in my weight. I was so overwhelmed by the size of the obstacle that I talked myself out of the journey before it even started.

## Make the Decision

The enemy keeps us stuck by diverting us from one very important truth: we don't have to do everything at once.

No one knows this better than sailors. They know that a big ship is turned just one degree at a time. To expect it to turn faster is insanity.

But I bought into that insanity in my life. I knew I was huge, but I still expected to be able to solve my problem overnight. And because I couldn't, I got discouraged and quit before I even started.

That's why hearing the dime story that New Year's Eve was so instrumental for me. Picking up one dime at a time and watching it all add up was so simple, yet so profound. I could see how it worked! My neighbors had coin jars filled with fifty, sixty, even one hundred dollars—all because they added to their collections one coin at a time.

Saint Francis of Assisi said it like this: "Start with what is necessary, then move to what is possible, and suddenly you will be doing the impossible."

If I had to even think of losing over 200 pounds, I wouldn't have begun the journey. I didn't need to do it all at once; I just needed to make the decision to start somewhere.

And frankly, many of us run from that. I know I did. What I didn't realize was that when I put off making a decision, I was actually making a decision. I was deciding to do nothing—to allow the status quo to continue. From there, the thoughts spiraled in one direction: down. No matter what your weight in sin, if you decide to do nothing, it's easy to think that you're a victim, that you are locked in, and that you can't do anything about your situation.

But there is something you can do. You can start somewhere: right where you are. Decide to take one tiny action. That decision, however small, starts a process that will change your life.

## Baby Steps, One Day at a Time

I spent years looking at my problem as one giant mountain to climb. It didn't occur to me that a mountain is climbed one step at a time. But that all changed when I heard about the dimes. And then when Jeff told me that I would make small changes to my eating and exercise one week at a time, everything started to make sense.

> **Week 0: Commit to ninety days.** *Can you do just ninety days?* I asked myself, knowing that Jeff wouldn't work with me unless I committed to stick it out for three months. *C'mon, dude. Just ninety days. If it doesn't work, you're off the hook.* I was desperate and scared, so I agreed.
>
> **Week 1: No fried foods.** I decided that I could do this for a week. Giving up fried foods didn't seem to be that big of a sacrifice. After all, there were plenty of other things to eat. It wasn't like Jeff was asking me to eliminate an entire food group. I could still eat bread and ice cream. After the first few days, I realized that I didn't miss fried foods like I had thought I would.
>
> **Week 2: Chicken and fish only.** In addition to avoiding fried foods, I cut out red meat. There was still plenty to eat. I was still satisfied after my meals. I didn't shrivel up and blow away. Actually, it wasn't that bad at all. In fact, I was thrilled to know that I was keeping these very

simple promises to myself after years and years of making—and breaking—the diet promise. Maybe I really could go all the way.

**Week 3: Walk fifteen minutes every other morning.** In week 3, while sticking to the small changes I'd made in my diet during the previous weeks, I added movement. I got up early to walk on my treadmill. Every other morning wasn't really that bad. Yes, I complained sometimes, but I did it.

**Week 4: Be mindful.** During the first three weeks, my breakfasts consisted of oatmeal, eggs, and toast with butter. "You might want to skip the butter you put on your bread," Jeff told me. And I listened. That same week a friend showed me how to make smoothies for breakfast. I made them with fruit, ice, and protein, and they tasted like ice cream. I was hooked. Ice cream for breakfast: it was a dream come true.

After four weeks, I realized that my mind-set was changing. I had always been great at starting things but not so good at finishing. But after doing it Jeff's way for a month, I felt different. I made one small change each week, which gave me seven days to actually do what I had promised to myself and Jeff. Knowing that I had been honest about my behavior gave me a new triumph to celebrate each day. It felt amazing.

I believe that the Lord wants us to live one day at a time. When He was creating the heavens and the earth, He paused for a moment at the end of each day, surveyed His work, and saw that it was good (see Genesis 1:4, 10, 12, 18, 21, 25).

God always took time to appreciate what He had

accomplished. He didn't step back, look around, and complain about what He had left to do. He didn't say, *Ugh! I only got half of the things on My to-do list done. I still have to create the sky, the oceans, the people, and the animals, not to mention the weather and everything else.* He had other days to finish the rest. He took things one day at a time and took time to savor His success at the end of the day. That's exactly how He wants us to live.

*Today Calvin didn't eat any fried foods. Today is good. Tomorrow there may be other things for him to work on, but for today, it's good. I'm going to work out his issue with debt. I'm going to work out his low self-esteem. But today I'm only asking him to make a healthy eating choice.*

Jeff continued to have me make small changes, and by ninety days, those small changes added up to visible results. Looking back, I can see that if I had tried to make all the changes at once—eliminating fried foods, red meat, butter on my toast—I would have failed. But making one small change each week and adding another change the following week wasn't hard at all.

## A God of Process

Jeff showed me that I could use that momentum to keep moving forward.

"It's changing your perspective and changing your mind," he told me. "If you lost only 5 pounds every ninety days, you still would lose 20 pounds at the end of the year. Do that for two more years, and you've lost 60 pounds."

As the weeks continued, I realized that my mind was slowly renewing. Through Jeff's guidance and the Spirit of the Lord, I could see that my thinking about weight loss was flawed. To me and many other obese people, losing 60 pounds in three years is unacceptable. It's too long to wait.

But that's not the way God thinks. We believe that it's all or nothing with the Lord, when in fact, that's the enemy's way of thinking. The enemy says we must change everything all at once to reach the goal as quickly as possible. To the enemy, diets are one-time events. They have a beginning and an end. You go on, and you go off. If you don't do it perfectly or if it takes too long, why try at all? If you do happen to make it to the end, you've earned the right to go back to the way you used to eat. Then it's just a matter of time before your old eating habits take you right back to where you started—typically with a 20-pound bonus.

Fortunately the Lord has very different ideas. God is the God of process. *It's not about the goal; it's about the journey,* He says. To our Creator, the process starts with a simple decision and an open mind. *Start somewhere,* says the Lord. *Start where you are, and start small.* Renewing our minds means allowing God to purge them of all the lies the enemy tells us about ourselves, our relationships with others, and the substances we abuse to "protect" ourselves from the slings and arrows of life.

People who don't use food as a sedative can easily see that weight loss is a process. They know that it simply requires eating less over time. Eventually the weight comes off. Obese people don't see the process, just the goal. Obese people get upset when the goal isn't achieved quickly and effortlessly. The enemy beats us up when we try to do it all at once and fail. If we can't have it all at once, then we won't try at all.

Focus on the goal, and the goal will elude you. Focus on the process, and lasting change will happen. The process revealed the truth about my character. Some of it was pretty, and some of it wasn't. I was insecure. I was afraid of rejection. I wanted to be accountable in my own way and on my own terms. But I also had a heart to help people.

Whether your desire is to lose weight, quit drinking, or stop some other self-destructive behavior, focusing on the goal without looking at the truth of your character makes relapse more than just likely. It makes relapse inevitable.

## More than a Song

"Start Somewhere" is more than just a saying. It's more than just a song. It's an anthem about the process.

The song didn't come directly from my weight-loss story; it came from my struggle to start a music career. I was finally in Nashville and I knew I could sing, but I hadn't done anything to make my dream come true. I didn't know the first thing about recording an album. I seemed stuck on dead center and couldn't get moving.

I called my friend Greg to talk, and when he picked up the phone, I could tell that something was troubling him. He told me that he was really down and discouraged. I could relate to his pain.

"You've just got to get up and get going," I told him. "Just get started . . . begin the journey."

A few days later I was talking to a songwriter about the challenges of getting a career started in the music industry. Okay, I was actually complaining about them.

"You've just got to start somewhere," he said.

And a lightbulb went on in my head. Start somewhere. It was the same advice I had given to Greg. The same advice I was following in my weight-loss process. And then the song just came to me.

*Life has you back in the same old place, feeling*
  *overwhelmed,*
*Telling yourself that you just can't win and doubting*
  *once again.*
*The door is open, embrace the moment, take a leap*
  *of faith.*
*Why are you waiting, got to start somewhere,*
*Nothing is changing until you start somewhere.*
*Freedom is calling, love will take you there.*
*But it's up to you to start somewhere.*

Nothing is going to change until you begin the process and take that first step. You can think about it and you can meditate on it, but until you take that first step, nothing is going to happen.

My first recording of the vocals for "Start Somewhere" was for a demo. When it was time to actually do the album, I didn't want to rerecord the vocal track because the original was such a perfect expression of my state of mind at the time. I was emotionally raw and overwhelmed with pain, all of which came out in the vocals. It was this authentic state that gave the song its power. That song became the springboard for my ministry.

Starting somewhere is about more than just feeling the emotions. It is about turning awareness into action. Millions of people are aware that they are overweight. Millions are aware that they are hooked on drugs or alcohol. Millions are aware that they suffer from lust. But they do nothing with that awareness—except maybe complain. *Isn't it sad that 65 percent of America is overweight? And isn't it sad about the divorce rate? By the way, will you pass the cake?*

Awareness is useless unless it's backed by action. And unless that action is connected to a goal, it's nothing more than wheel-spinning. But as we've already seen, simply having a goal isn't enough. Being willing to focus on a goal while being open to what you might learn about yourself during the journey is what really matters. It wasn't the loss of 215 pounds that changed me; it was the process of discovering who I was during the journey that brought about the real change. It was . . .

> Waking up in the morning and telling myself, *I'm going to do this just for today* and actually following through on my commitment

> Not seeing the numbers change as quickly as I would have liked—in spite of working hard and being honest about what I ate—but continuing anyway

> Being nervous about what life would be like at a normal weight and still sticking to my eating and exercise plan

> Allowing myself to be vulnerable in front of people so they could know my story, which meant risking their disapproval or rejection

> Realizing that God had allowed me to reach this point in order to use my story to help others

The process forced me to confront the real truth about myself in every area of life. But most of all, it forced me to admit that the goal didn't really matter all that much. Getting to a certain weight wasn't as important as what I learned during the journey to reach that number.

## The Lesson Is in the Journey

The children of Israel had a similar situation. They were enslaved in Egypt, and things were getting worse. Moses said it was time to go, but many of the people didn't want to leave until they knew where they were going. They had questions—lots of questions—and they wanted assurances before they were ready to pack up and leave. Maybe the conversation went like this:

> **Average joes:** What do you mean, you want us to leave Egypt? Yeah, we're slaves and all, but at least we know what each new day will bring.

> **Moses:** The only thing that you need to know is that it's time to go.

> **Average joes:** But it's not so bad here. What is all this talk of the Promised Land? Where is it? How will we get there? What will we eat on the way? Are there any roadside rests? Do you have a map? What about bathroom facilities?

> **Moses:** Look, this may not make a lot of sense at the moment, but you're going to have to trust me that you will be better off outside of Egypt than you are inside of Egypt. I've got GPS (God Positioning System) version 1 that will be guiding us.

> **Average joes:** We're not going until we have a detailed itinerary.

> **Moses (fuming):** Come on! Just walk through the door!

I have always felt sorry for Moses. What a job he had! Getting the Hebrews to do anything must have been like herding cats. He listened to so much whining, complaining, and carping, it's a wonder he didn't lose his temper much sooner. He was dealing with the same thing then that God has to deal with in us every day. We know that the things we want to achieve are possible, but we focus on the obstacles, the questions, and the what-ifs.

It was like that for me with my first album. I didn't even know if I should do an album. What if only ten people heard it? What if no one cared? I blazed forward anyway. When I was recording the album, God answered my questions. *If it's for ten people, it's still ten people. If it's for 10 million, then it's for 10 million, but it's not your job to worry about that.*

I was capable of recording an album. Anyone is. Anyone, that is, who wants to record his or her voice and give the recording to others to enjoy. But some of us won't even make the first move because of all the unanswered questions: How am I going to get it distributed? Who is going to produce it?

In my case, it took a friend and a verbal two-by-four to get me back on track. "You're worried about who is going to produce and distribute this album, and you don't even have any songs," he said. "Start writing songs!"

I hated hearing it, but he was right. I wanted answers. I wanted all the what-ifs to be resolved before even starting. Sometimes God just wants us to shut up, walk through the door, and leave the destination management to Him.

## Get Off Dead Center

There are a lot of people out there who got themselves off dead center and started somewhere. Oprah Winfrey is a good example. She was going to school for journalism, and she got a call one day from a TV station to become an anchor. At first she considered turning down the offer. After all, she had to finish college. But her professor encouraged her to take the opportunity.

"Are you crazy?" he asked. "You need to take this job. People go to school so they can get those kinds of jobs, and one falls into your lap right now. This is a chance for you to begin the process of being what you wanted all along. This is your moment."

Oprah left school and seized the moment, and the rest is history. Today she holds honorary degrees from some of the most esteemed universities in the nation.

Please don't get me wrong. My goal isn't to discourage people from going to school. My goal is to encourage you to recognize when the Lord is prompting you to take the first step on your journey. When you have the chance to start somewhere, don't put off the decision because you see too many obstacles in your way. Don't put it off because you have questions that you can't answer. Just start somewhere. Move.

That first step will vary for different people. If alcohol is your issue, starting somewhere might mean going to an Alcoholics Anonymous meeting. If you're having trouble in your marriage, you might visit a marriage counselor or your pastor. No matter what your issue, three things will help you turn your awareness into action.

**Talk about it.** Getting off dead center often starts by sharing your thoughts with someone. Make a public commitment. Enlist support from others. Tell a friend what you're working on and when you have completed it. Many of us take the commitments we make to others more seriously than the promises we make only to our-selves. At the very least, going public with your inten-tions makes it more difficult to avoid your goal in secret.

**Get feedback.** Talking to another person forces you to organize your thoughts. Once your goal is out in the open, you may hear that you are attempting too much. A plan that seemed overwhelming in your mind might seem more feasible as you explain it to a listener. The Lord speaks through others, so listen carefully to feed-back from people you respect and trust.

**Avoid comparisons.** Before I started working on my record, I spent a lot of time listening to recordings by great artists. I was listening for inspiration, but I found myself feeling discouraged instead. *I can't do that,* I told myself after listening to one particularly gifted singer. *He's way too good. Way too polished. There's no way I can ever measure up to that.*

A friend pointed out the error in my reasoning. "Calvin," he said, "you are comparing your first album to that artist's eighth album. Go easy on yourself."

He was right. This album was my beginning. It was my first. Just as the artist I admired so much had improved with every album, so would I.

God says that He orders your steps. He doesn't want you to be stuck. He doesn't want you to be covered up by your weight in sin. He wants you to decide to take that small first step. We are who we are and we are where we are because of choices we've made. Deciding to do nothing is making a choice. What will you choose today?

CHAPTER 8

# STEP 6: ELIMINATE THE EXCUSES

WHAT'S YOUR EXCUSE for not laying down your weight in sin?

I don't have time to go to the gym.

I know somebody who's in worse shape than I am.

I deserve a splurge once in a while.

I have affairs to save my marriage.

I drink because my job is so stressful.

My pot smoking doesn't hurt anyone.

Before my weight-loss journey, I used every excuse in the book not to lose weight. *I still look cool. I may be big, but I'm not sloppy big. I still have friends.*

During my weight-loss journey, I found reasons to resist following Jeff's instructions. *I have to be at work at 8 a.m. There's no time to walk on the treadmill.*

My tendency to make excuses persists to this day. *I can't work out when I'm on the road. Hotels don't have good gyms. It's impossible to make good eating choices when I'm traveling. How do you eat healthy in an airport?*

For me, making excuses is as easy as breathing. Maybe it's the same for you.

## Rebellion in Disguise

From the beginning, God established clear boundaries around human behavior. He did this for our protection. These boundaries aren't a bunch of rules meant to make our lives miserable or to keep us from having fun. They are the user's manual delivered straight from the manufacturer, designed by our Creator so we can live our lives safely and securely inside His will for us.

If you read the user's manual for any electrical appliance, one of the first things you'll notice is the caution not to immerse the plugged-in appliance in water. If you do, there are consequences.

It's the same for us. Violate God's boundaries, and you'll face the consequences.

Adam and Eve are the poster children for broken boundaries. God gave them only one boundary, and they blew it.

*Everything I made in the Garden is yours for the taking . . . except this one little thing,* He told them. *Just don't eat this one little thing.*

We all know what happened next. Thanks to a little serpentine persuasion, Adam and Eve decided that the rules didn't apply to them. And after the defiance came the excuses.

*But the serpent told me it was okay.*

*That woman You sent made me do it.*

There were probably other excuses that got cut from the official version of the story.

*It's not fair that we can have everything else and not the fruit of the tree of knowledge.*

*Why did You put it right in front of our noses unless You really wanted us to have it?*

*I was hungry, but I didn't have time to walk over to the pear tree and have a snack. This tree was so much closer.*

*I thought the serpent was speaking for You. You mean You didn't send him?*

No matter what the excuses were, God didn't want to hear them. God had given Adam and Eve everything they needed—freedom, joy, innocence, plenty of food, a beautiful place to live—and asked them not to do this one little thing. Yet they did it, made excuses, and hid. And then, with a giant thud, the consequences fell into place. And here we are.

Violating boundaries is rebellion, and we use excuses to justify that rebellion. Just as a fish dies if it is removed from the water, we, too, will experience death if we push past our boundaries. In our case, death comes in the form of separation from God. It was true in the Garden, and it's true in our lives today. Whether we violate God's boundaries willfully and defiantly or slyly and quietly, pushing the envelope sentences us to a life cut off from the only power that can make us whole. There's no way to escape the consequences, no matter how complicated or reasonable our rationalizations may seem.

Maybe you're rationalizing right now.

*What Adam and Eve did was stupid,* you think. *They ate the fruit, and the world went down the tubes. But my situation is different. My porn addiction isn't going to result in the damnation of humankind for all eternity. It's not hurting anybody—it's just a little harmless pleasure. After all, I work hard and don't ask for much. At least I'm not visiting prostitutes.*

The future of humankind may not be hanging in the balance, but the future of your soul, your serenity, and your relationships most definitely are.

There was nowhere for Adam and Eve to hide, and there's nowhere for us to hide. God's boundaries are immovable, and they are there for our protection. If we had observed these boundaries, our natural instincts might not have spiraled out of control, leading us to all sorts of addictions, obsessions, and compulsions that have clogged our direct line to God and sentenced us to emotional, spiritual, and physical death.

Physical death from your addiction may come quickly, or it may come slowly. If you're a junkie who craves the heroin high, your death may come quietly as you overdose in a dark corner or a back alley. Or it may come violently when you're murdered by a deranged drug dealer. If you're a sex addict, your death may come slowly in the form of AIDS or brutally from the beatings that inmates reserve for child molesters. If you're a compulsive eater, death may come slowly as your worn-out pancreas struggles to produce insulin or abruptly when your oxygen-starved heart seizes up. No matter when you take your last breath, your spiritual death will happen much earlier if you are living far outside of God's will.

## End the Blame Game

Rebellion may be human nature, but the enemy doesn't have to have the last word. No matter how we have let our natural instincts run wild, we never lose the power to choose what to do next. We *can* set boundaries and choose to live a life without excuses; it's just difficult to see how sometimes.

So what can we do?

**Ask God to help.** Whatever brings spiritual death to you must be cut out of your life. For most of us, we can't do this on our own. We need supernatural assistance from a God who steps in to help us only when we are absolutely certain we can't do it ourselves. If we have surrendered the problem to God, He gives us the power we need to choose *not* to engage in our destructive behaviors.

People who have admitted that they can't do it themselves get their "chooser" restored. A recovering alcoholic can choose to avoid bars or choose not to associate with former binge-drinking buddies. A recovering sex addict can choose to cut off contact with an affair partner or people who aren't friends of his marriage. A recovering food addict can choose not to take that first bite of a food that triggers a full-blown binge. A recovering porn addict can choose not to have a computer in the house.

Asking for and receiving God's help assumes that you have a relationship with Him in the first place. If you don't have a relationship or you feel that He is miles away, your ability to make good choices will be compromised. In my case, the boundaries around what I put in my mouth need to be airtight. If my boundaries are porous or I'm in a bad place spiritually, I lose the ability to choose.

**Know yourself.** Some people may be able to handle having a doughnut for breakfast. Not me. Left to my own devices, I will try to fill the God-shaped hole in my soul with baked goods. One doughnut, just one, starts a chain reaction of chewing that eventually robs me of my power of choice and leaves me covered with powdered sugar and sprinkles. It's like a runaway train. One doughnut will lead to five, which will lead to a dozen. And the destruction doesn't stop there. Since I blew it with the doughnuts, I figure I might as well have all the other foods I like so much and haven't had in a long time. After all, today is shot. I'll just get back on the wagon tomorrow. But of course, tomorrow never comes. Once I pick up something outside of my defined eating plan, I'm off to the races.

Today, however, I know how that story ends, and I don't try to convince myself that this time will be different. Given that knowledge, I can choose not to allow the story to begin in the first place, instead asking the Lord for the answer to the real problem.

**Get off the pity pot.** My denial of basic truths about myself and my secret wish that things could be different used to keep me from setting and sticking to boundaries. Even today, there are times when I really wish that I could be like everyone else. I want to be a normal eater, someone who can have a doughnut here and there. I want to be someone who can walk into a room, see a box of cookies, enjoy a few bites of a cookie, set it down, get focused on something else, and come back three hours later to find the half-eaten cookie still on the plate. But that's not me. I'm the person who eats one and immediately starts plotting how I can have the rest without anyone noticing that I have eaten them all.

Why should I be the only one who can't enjoy all

those sweet holiday foods? Why should I be the one who always has to have less than he wants? Why can't I be a normal eater?

This whining is dangerous. Wishing things were different reveals a basic lack of acceptance of the lessons God has put in my path to help develop my character. Wishing for an alternate reality is a roadblock in the path to living within God's will.

**Develop new habits.** Jeff told me that it takes about twenty-one days of doing something to make that new behavior a habit. That's just three weeks, which isn't really all that long when you think about it. Since I had so many bad habits, I had a lot of work to do. Walking on the treadmill became a new habit for me. I had all sorts of reasons not to do it, but I exercised my power of choice. I eliminated the excuses by going to bed an hour earlier so I could get up at 5:30 a.m. to walk. Working out while on the road was another habit I had to develop. Instead of complaining that hotels didn't have good gyms, I went outside to walk. It didn't kill me!

**Compensate with positive behaviors.** Bingeing on sweets was a bad habit I knew I needed to stop. Though I couldn't see myself giving up sweets for the rest of my life, I knew that I could enjoy them once in a while if I canceled out the treat with a different, more positive behavior. In my case, it was a workout. If I'm working out on a regular basis, then I can afford an occasional indulgence.

**Lean on accountability partners.** We have already talked about the role accountability partners can play in keeping you focused on your goal. Friends, family, and personal trainers can really help you cut through the excuses and keep you moving forward.

The bottom line is simple. When it comes to laying down your weight in sin, there is no such thing as a good excuse. Sure, there may be hardships in your life. Living and working on the road was a hardship that made it tough for me to exercise and eat right. Not having enough money in my checking account was a hardship that made me want to avoid opening my credit card statements when they arrived in the mail. Being teased as a child was a hardship that made me want to sedate myself with excess food.

Difficult circumstances will always exist, requiring us to make the choice to live within the boundaries God has set for us. Jesus told us that we would face hardships (see John 16:33) and that they would draw us closer to Him. So why do we use those hardships as justification to live outside His will for us? We may have a misguided expectation that life should be easy. But it's not. And that's no excuse for making excuses.

## The Mother of All Excuses

We've already talked about how trainers can serve as accountability partners. I feel very strongly about the role of my trainer in my journey, so I want to come back to this issue.

I can't stress enough how important it is to rely on a personal trainer to help you lose weight. A good personal trainer will help you stop making excuses—that is, if you can get past the biggest excuse of all, the excuse that most people deliver in a whiny voice while feeling massive amounts of self-pity: "But I can't afford a trainer!" (sniffle, sob, gasp).

Okay, so you're on a tight budget. I was too, but after some serious soul-searching, I realized that I always seemed to have money to pay for the foods I wanted.

Next to being willing to surrender the very big problem of my weight to the Lord, hiring a personal trainer was the single most important thing I did to jump-start my weight-loss journey. I want to help you do the math so you can see for yourself that you can't afford *not* to get professional help to lift this weight in sin. Let's say that a session with a personal trainer costs $50 a session. Let's say you need the trainer three days a week. That's $150 per week and roughly $600 per month.

Before you start hyperventilating, stay with me. We're going to look at where your money is currently going and cut through all the excuses that are keeping you stuck.

Let's start with your eating habits.

How many times do you eat in restaurants each week? I'm talking about places where you go in, sit down, and order. Every day? Three times a day? Ten times a week? More? Write the number on a piece of paper. What is the average cost of a restaurant meal? Take some time to think about all the different places you go, and calculate the average cost per meal. Write the amount under the first number. Now multiply the number of meals by the average cost. What is your weekly total?

What do you spend on groceries each week? This includes everything you bring home, including the lettuce, vegetables, and fruits that end up rotting in the crisper when you blow your diet. Write your grocery total on the same piece of paper.

How many times each week do you go through fast-food drive-throughs? Don't forget to include the times you go through the same drive-through more than once a day hoping that shift change will have occurred so you won't be recognized. Write the number on your paper. How much do you spend in the average trip through the drive-through? Multiply the number of drive-through trips by the average cost. What is your weekly total?

How many times a day do you stop by stores, restaurants, or bakeries to buy snacks that you'll take home to binge on in private? This includes items that you tell the checkout clerk you are buying for others but intend to devour yourself (in secret, of course). Write the number on your paper. How much do you spend per day on those foods? Write down the amount. Multiply the number of trips by the average cost. What's your weekly total? Add up all the weekly totals.

Now I dare you to tell me that you don't have at least some money you can divert from your food budget each week to a session with a personal trainer. Even if you just give up your snack trips, you will free up some cash that could go for personal training. If money is so tight that you still can't afford a personal trainer, join a local gym and get involved in group fitness classes. If you are really serious about wanting to surrender this weight in sin, you will make it happen.

When I want something, no one can stop me from getting it. Right now I want a grand piano. I want it, and I'm going to get it. There's just one little obstacle. This grand piano costs $3,500—on sale. It's expensive and I don't have the money today, but I'm going to move heaven and earth to save the money for it because it is a priority for me. I will work harder, sell more CDs, and make more stops on my tour. I will get it, and I will pay cash.

When you want something so badly that it becomes a priority in your life, the excuses will just fall away.

## Behind the Curtain of Excuses

If you still can't find your way to a personal trainer or even to a gym, maybe a little digging is in order to find out what's fueling the excuses. Is it fear? Are you afraid of what people will think if they see a fat person at the gym? I know I was.

Think about it. Isn't the gym where you would expect to find fat people trying to get in shape? It makes sense to the thin, slightly overweight, and flabby people you'll find on the treadmills, elliptical trainers, and rowing machines. But to people who are obese, this logic makes no sense at all. They don't see that others at the gym are there to work on their own fitness programs; they believe they are there to silently mock all the fat people!

A friend of mine once shared a story that makes this point beautifully. She is a compulsive overeater who has spent years of recovery in a twelve-step program that requires weighed and measured meals, extensive work with an accountability partner, and abstinence from addictive foods. You would never know that she has lost 90 pounds and has kept it off for fourteen years. She looks like a normal-size person. Anyway, my friend was serving as an accountability partner to an obese woman who kept relapsing. A major cause of the woman's relapses was her resistance to using a food scale to measure portions when eating in restaurants. "I am so uncomfortable using the scale in public," whined the obese woman. "I don't want other people to look at me and think I have an eating disorder."

"Darling," replied my friend, "look in the mirror. You are the size of a house. Everyone already knows you have an eating disorder."

Underneath the obese woman's excuse was a paralyzing self-obsession actively encouraged by our old "friend," the enemy.

*Everyone is looking at you,* whispers the enemy. *They're all just too polite to let on. They think you're a freak. And you are!* This self-centered fear led her to believe that she was the focal point of every diner in the room, when in truth, hardly anyone was looking. This distorted thinking knocked her off balance every time, which led to food choices in restaurants that almost inevitably ended in a binge.

Many excuses are rooted in our self-centered fear of loss—of money, status, or a perceived advantage.

*What if I can't pay my bills and have to file bankruptcy and my name is in the paper?*

*What if I admit my affairs and my wife decides to leave me?*

*What if people see me going into the church where the AA meeting is held and they think I'm an alcoholic?*

These fruitless what-if statements are part of the standard operating procedure for the enemy in his plan to keep us disconnected from God. Trust me here. I know what I'm talking about, because I have tried all these excuses to avoid making positive changes in my life. But excuses just keep you stuck.

If you are serious about turning your weight in sin over to the Lord, you will be given a precious gift: the restoration of your power of choice. You will have the ability to recognize excuses for what they are: elaborate justifications for subtle—and not-so-subtle—rebellion against God's boundaries for right living. What will you choose today?

# CHAPTER 9

# STEP 7: ACCEPT THE NEED FOR TRAINING WHEELS

REMEMBER WHAT IT WAS LIKE the first time you rode a bicycle?

Were you nervous? Were you afraid that you couldn't balance on two wheels?

I was.

As a three-year-old, I watched the older kids zoom around on their bicycles. They banked their turns and popped wheelies. They made it look easy. But I wasn't so sure.

When my parents brought home my first bicycle, I was terrified. Now it was my turn to swoop around corners and pop wheelies. But I was afraid to even get on.

They seemed to sense my fear. "I bought these to help you out," said my father, holding up two metal bars with black wheels at each end.

I watched as he bolted the training wheels to the rear frame of my bike. "These will save you from a lot of skinned knees until you get the hang of balancing," said my mother as my father tightened the last bolt. "You won't need these little guys forever. Just let us know when you're ready to try riding without them. There's no hurry."

I remember feeling great relief. Though I was afraid of falling and getting hurt, I really did want to learn. The training wheels would make it easier. I felt safe knowing that they would be there to catch me if I leaned too far to the left or the right. So I rode and rode, trying as best as I could to imitate the big guys. I couldn't bank my turns, but I was able to eke out a few wheelies. The training wheels were working! They were making me ride! Zooming around the neighborhood, intoxicated by my newfound freedom, I grew more confident.

Before long, I started to realize that I hardly ever felt the training wheels touch the ground when I rode. Could it be that I was balancing on two wheels? Even for a few seconds? It was a scary thought. I was certain that the training wheels were the reason I was able to ride. The thought of riding without them filled me with anxiety. *I'm going to keep these forever,* I promised myself.

But my parents had other ideas. They had been watching my progress and felt I was ready to try riding without the training wheels. "I'm not sure I can do it," I pleaded. "I'm scared. What if I fall?"

My heart was in my throat as I watched my father unbolt the training wheels. This was terrible. I couldn't do it. I was sure I would fall. Those training wheels were the reason I could have so much fun. But my parents insisted. "You're ready, Son," said my father, steadying the freestanding bicycle so I could climb on.

After I was in the seat, he gave me and the bicycle a push. "Pedal," he said. "You already know what to do. Just ride like you always have, just like you would if the wheels were on."

I pedaled. The bike wobbled, but I was moving. And then, just like that, something clicked. I was balancing. I was riding. *I know how to do this!* I thought as I pedaled away. *I am doing this!*

## Training Wheels Unlock Potential

Most healthy young children have the ability to ride a bike. The skills needed to balance, turn, stop, start, and react are all present. The potential is there. It's just that the child doesn't realize it. Training wheels prop a child up physically and emotionally until the child realizes that he or she can do it alone.

One day about a year into my training with Jeff, I recalled the experience of learning to ride a bike. "Working with you is like having training wheels for my life," I told him. It's just that my training wheels looked like Sylvester Stallone!

On my bike, training wheels kept me from teetering too far in one direction. They kept me balanced. They kept me focused on learning the skills I needed to ride by removing the distraction of fear.

In my life, following Jeff's workout instructions to the letter kept me on track while I practiced new and unfamiliar ways of eating, moving, and dealing with my emotions. Like many obese people, I was caught in a trap of all-or-nothing thinking that often led to extreme behaviors. Left to my own devices, this all-or-nothing thinking led to actions that were totally out of balance.

*Why can't I be normal?* I often asked myself, but the truth was I didn't really know what normal meant. "Normal is a cycle on a washing machine," a friend once told me.

The concept of *enough* was just as foreign. If one was good, more was better. Somehow my way of responding to life was way out of balance. I was living on the edge of excess. Nothing in my life was normal.

I wasn't a normal eater. I wanted to be thin, but I wanted to eat everything.

I wasn't a normal exerciser. I wanted to be buff, but I didn't want to work out.

I wasn't a normal consumer. I wanted to have more of everything so I would look affluent, but I didn't have money.

I wasn't a normal debtor. I wanted to max out my credit cards but ignore my bills.

This all changed when I worked with Jeff. He kept me focused on all the things I needed to be doing to lose weight. My tendency was to exercise compulsively without addressing my desire to overeat. He kept me balanced by bringing my attention back to both issues. Without him, I would have promised to work out and then broken the promise or, even worse, worked out too hard and burned out, quitting out of sheer exhaustion or injury. Without him, I would have tried to make massive changes to my diet all at once and then quit out of frustration at the first slipup.

My problem was that I was trying to get God to surrender to me. I was trying to impose my insatiable will—the desire for more food, more money, more things, more recognition, more status, and more fame—on a God who wanted nothing more than for me to put down the fork and let Him run my life. As I continued to work with Jeff, I could see that he was propping me up physically, mentally, and emotionally. He was protecting me from my deeply ingrained all-or-nothing way of responding to life until new habits could be formed.

Admitting that I didn't have all the answers and being open to following Jeff's instructions was a form of surrender that was

new to me. For years I had really believed that I had surrendered my life to the Lord, but now I could see that I had always
held back in the area of my weight. And honestly, there were
other areas too. Instead of having no willpower, I could see that
I had plenty. My will—my desire to have whatever I wanted
whenever I wanted it—was the problem. I didn't need more
willpower; I needed less!

Jeff was training more than my body. He was literally training
my will. Under the guidance of this messenger sent straight from
the Lord, I learned to surrender my will, find my balance, and discover my unlimited potential for positive change. I began to open
myself to new ways of thinking, new ways of behaving, and new
ways of reacting to life's triumphs and tragedies. I found myself
replacing old self-defeating thoughts with new positive ones.

"What you think about, you bring about," Jeff told me. At
the same time, with his gentle encouragement, I tried on new
behaviors for size. "You can't think your way into right acting,"
he would say. "But you can act your way into right thinking."

These new ways of thinking and acting were uncharted terri-
tory for me. Every time I got up to exercise without Jeff having
to call and remind me was the spiritual equivalent of riding my
bike without the training wheels touching the ground. Every
time I allowed Jeff to talk me into completing my workout
when I wanted to quit was the spiritual equivalent of the training wheels catching me as I teetered too far to the left. Every
time I got discouraged and wanted to throw in the towel because
I wasn't seeing results fast enough and Jeff encouraged me to
look at things differently, it was the spiritual equivalent of the
training wheels catching me as I leaned too far to the right.

Eventually I started to realize that the ability to correct
myself before teetering too far off balance—with my food, my

exercise, my emotions, my responses to life—had always been in me. Working with Jeff just helped me see it.

## Training Your Will

Are there areas of your life where you feel like you could use a good pair of training wheels?

Recommitting to your marriage

Getting your weight under control

Sticking to a fitness program

Reducing out-of-control spending

Getting off pills, booze, or drugs

Ending an addictive relationship

Giving up the smokes once and for all

What will your training wheels look like? Who or what will . . .

help you face the truth that your weight in sin is blocking you from the peaceful, joy-filled life that the Lord wants you to have?

keep your thoughts and actions on track as you make the decision to shed your weight in sin and try on new thoughts and behaviors for size?

hold your hand as the enemy tries to convince you that life without your weight in sin will be a humorless, unbearable existence?

catch you when you feel like crumbling from the paralyzing fear of failure?

encourage you as you face the inevitable setbacks and challenges?

help you surrender your weight in sin once and for all and allow the Holy Spirit to work in your life, unlocking your potential for self-discipline and excellence?

What will it take for you to make lasting, positive lifestyle changes on your own? What will life be like when you let go of those training wheels?

The Lord is on standby for us at all times. Jesus called on Him right before He gave His life for us.

*Father, if you are willing, please take this cup of suffering away from me. Yet I want your will to be done, not mine.*
—LUKE 22:42

Though it wasn't easy, Jesus knew what He was called to do, and He surrendered His will to God's will.

Heartfelt surrender is the first step for us as well. Surrender opens the door for God's power to work in your life. What training wheels will God send to help you gain confidence in your ability to release your weight in sin?

If you have a lot of weight to lose, your training wheels may come in the form of a personal trainer or a nutritional counselor. Training wheels might be an overeaters' support group that helps you address the emotional drivers of your eating habits. These habits train your will to be a good steward of your physical body.

If you are in financial trouble, your training wheels may come in the form of a church group or an accountability partnership designed to help people rein in spending. Training wheels may involve sitting down with your spouse or a close friend who helps you cut up credit cards, set up payment plans with creditors, and transition your financial life to an all-cash envelope system. These habits train your will to live within your means.

If you are hooked on pornography, your training wheels may come in the form of moving your computer into an open area of your house—say, the kitchen or family room—where others can freely look over your shoulder when you're online. Training wheels may also involve confessing your addiction to your spouse and agreeing to counseling to address underlying psychological issues. These habits train your will to respect boundaries and say no to inappropriate content.

If you are ensnared in an inappropriate relationship, your training wheels may come in the form of a no-contact letter that formally ends the relationship. It may also include disclosure of the affairs to your spouse, complete transparency, and a commitment to individual or marital counseling. These habits train your will to focus your energies on healing your marriage.

Note that every example of training wheels involves at least one other person. This is no accident. God does some of His best work through other people. There's nothing like admitting your struggles to another human being to prove that you are willing to finally accept God's help.

It was the same for me when I was young. The trust I had in my father when he bolted the training wheels to my bike—and when he took the wheels off again—was complete. I surrendered to the guidance he offered. God calls us to be like little children when it comes to trusting Him to manage every aspect of our lives. Are you ready to trust God to give you the training wheels you need?

## From Training Wheels to Training Wills

The insights I gained about my willfulness and my inner capacity for change were so profound that I built a ministry around them. The ministry was called Training Wills. An alternative to traditional fitness programs, which typically ignore the mental, emotional, and spiritual aspects of personal fitness, Training Wills was designed to help people just like me: everyday people who had tried—and failed—to make lasting, positive lifestyle changes on their own.

I wanted the ministry to focus on physical, emotional, and spiritual transformation through education, encouragement, and accountability—personal revival. As a conduit for the transformational powers of Jesus Christ, Training Wills was built to help people deepen their dependence on Christ and surrender strongholds that once seemed insurmountable.

No matter what your weight in sin, God has given you the ability to overcome it. It's just a matter of unlocking potential—training your will—with training wheels that keep you balanced and focused on the Source of your power.

What training wheels will you use to unlock your potential for change today?

# CHAPTER 10

# STEP 8: PERSEVERE TO THE END

BEGINNINGS ARE EASY. Endings can be glorious.

What about the middle? How do you survive the middle to arrive at the end?

When I started my weight-loss journey, I couldn't bear to think about the middle or the end. I needed to focus on the beginning, and every ninety days was a new one.

Eventually those ninety-day commitments added up. That's when I realized that I was no longer in the beginning. I was somewhere between the middle and the end. Instead of being excited, I was a bit worried.

*I've got to keep it going,* I thought. I was about a year into my weight-loss journey. I didn't want to embarrass myself or the Lord by failing.

The closer I got to my goal weight, the stronger these fears became. Would I actually reach my goal? Could I keep it going after I got there?

Always on standby, the enemy saw his opportunity.

*Calvin,* the enemy whispered, *do you really think you can keep doing this? You've been dieting for a year. You've lost 150 pounds. You've gone far enough. You're done. Why not enjoy some of those treats you've been denying yourself for so long? Just one won't hurt.*

Jeff had warned me to expect these thoughts. "The longer the race, the harder it gets," he told me. "The enemy will try even harder to knock you off balance."

After a year of following Jeff's instructions, my physical transformation was dramatic. My thinking had changed. I had a new willingness to surrender this part of my life to the Lord. But as I approached my goal weight, somehow I knew the honeymoon was over. I had been riding the pink cloud of excitement, buoyed by the realization that this time I was actually losing weight. There was actually a chance that I could be the thin person I had always dreamed I could be. But still I was nervous. Everything God had in store for me—my music career, especially—was dependent upon being successful at the one thing I had never been able to do before. Could I really keep it going?

## Don't Quit Five Minutes before the Miracle

Why do so many overweight people who diet successfully abandon their diets before they reach their goal weight? Sometimes impatience is the culprit. It was definitely an issue for me. After a year of dieting, my weight loss had slowed. Glaciers seemed speedy in comparison. I was discouraged.

Jeff stepped up my workout program. We did strenuous strength training three days a week, and I walked and jogged on the off days. I followed his food recommendations to the letter. Still the loss was slow.

CALVIN NOWELL ▶ 125

The next six months crept by. The enemy shifted into high gear. *Calvin,* the enemy shouted, seeing that his whispers weren't having the desired effect, *those ninety-day segments are just mind games. What about the five-year plan for your career? God said to lose the weight first, and you've done that. When do you start your real life and quit piddling your days away in a gym?*

I shared my fears with Jeff. "Losing the second 50 pounds is harder than losing the first 50," he assured me. "The second 100 will be harder than the first 100. The closer you get to your goal, the more grit you will need."

Grits? I immediately perked up. My mind was a bad neighborhood.

As my goal weight hovered just out of reach, temptation was everywhere. But there was something in me that wanted to keep fighting. I wanted to surrender to the Lord's plan for me so I could claim victory in His name. I worked harder, and I spent more time in the Word. I found all sorts of examples that reminded me that once you get past the early seasons of effort, diligent follow-through is essential until the goal is reached. This verse really stood out for me:

*If we endure hardship, we will reign with him.*
—2 TIMOTHY 2:12

I once heard a pastor say it this way: "Keep struggling, but just don't quit. Keep fighting! Wrestle with the Lord. When you give up and quit, you lose."

My weight loss wasn't a sprint. It wasn't a marathon either, at least not the 26.2-mile kind. My weight loss was an ultramarathon, one of those 100-mile races that really crazy people run.

So there I was, within sight of the finish line of my personal weight-loss marathon, and I was fading. Could I keep going? I had always believed in a strong finish. But there I was, in the last lap of the race, ready to quit! It was like watching a movie where the main character is trying to get something done, but it's difficult, and he's discouraged and ready to give up. You know that he is millimeters away from success, and you want to scream, "C'mon, dude! If you knew what was on the other side, you wouldn't even think this is an obstacle."

That was me. I felt like crying, screaming, and kicking. But I was determined to stick with it.

## Arriving at the Destination

At the end of those six months—eighteen months into my weight-loss journey—I finally hit my goal: 250 pounds—not a bad weight for a man who is six foot four. It was June 2004.

*I should feel great,* I thought after stepping off the scale. *I should be excited.* And part of me was. But something else was going on.

As I surveyed my body in the mirror, I realized that while I was happy to have achieved my goal weight, I wasn't content. Where was that buff body I secretly longed for? Where was that gorgeous hunk of a man who would be so irresistible to women? Where was the satisfaction of knowing that after so much sacrifice and deprivation it was all worth it because I was finally, completely, and totally *hot*?

The longer I looked at my image in the mirror, the more I realized that there was still much work to be done. Here I was, living my dream . . . but facing the reality that I still wouldn't want to be seen without a shirt. It was like someone had deflated a balloon, only the balloon was me.

It's hard for me to convey the mixed emotions I felt as I stared at my reflection. Yes, I was happy. But where was the satisfaction? I had started this journey thinking that once I saw the magic number on the scale, all the years of hating the way I looked would simply melt away. What I felt instead was a vague feeling of discontent. Had my entire journey been for this?

I felt like I had been on a train for eighteen months. The train stopped at a station, so I stepped out of my railcar onto the platform and looked around. This wasn't my stop! Yes, my ticket stub said this was where I was supposed to get off, but I was certain there had been a mistake. I had arrived at the weight I had dreamed about for years, but things didn't look or feel right.

I shared my concerns with Jeff. "It takes time—more than a year in some cases—for body mass to redistribute after a major weight loss," he said. "If your weight stays stable and you keep working out, your body will take care of this on its own. You can't rush it."

His words were small comfort. I wanted to be buff. I wanted to look like a bodybuilder.

Despite my feelings of discontent, I continued to follow Jeff's instructions and immersed myself in God's Word. Almost immediately, the Lord blessed me with new motivation to keep going, showing me that I could use the story of my journey to help others. I was going to become the poster child for healthy living after extreme weight loss. I was certain that I could look better. I just needed to work harder.

I fasted. I doubled up my workouts. I weighed myself every day. The number hovered around 250 pounds, just where I wanted it. And then the questions started.

"Man, are you sick?" asked a friend.

"Don't you think you've taken this a bit too far?" said another.

Their questions made me stop and think. Did I really look sick? Were they just jealous because I was able to lose weight and they couldn't? Might there be a grain of truth in their comments?

After two weeks of working out like a maniac, eating next to nothing, and feeling deprived all the time, I realized that the joy in the journey was gone. This wasn't fun anymore, and I wasn't sure why. I felt hollow.

I turned to God in prayer. His answer surprised me.

*Maybe you've got the wrong number.*

Could it be that 250 pounds wasn't the right weight for me? Should my maintaining weight be higher?

I resisted the notion. The Training Wills ministry was taking off, and I was making personal appearances in churches and telling my story. People were inspired. I felt like I needed to work harder to be what I thought others expected me to be.

And then, finally, it dawned on me. The enemy was back and trying to sneak in through a side door. *If you're leading a weight-loss ministry, you have to look the part,* the enemy said. *You have to be buff, sexy, and thin.* I could almost see the enemy flexing his devil biceps.

The enemy had taken my desire for approval and turned it on me, even in my success. He wanted to take my accomplishment and wring the Lord right out of it. The enemy wanted me frustrated, disappointed, and exiled from the only Power capable of helping me.

Something had to change. It was time to get back to reality. My original goal had never been to look like a bodybuilder. I was just a regular guy who needed to lose a couple of hundred pounds.

Trying to maintain an artificially low weight for my frame and height wasn't just unhealthy, it actually set the stage for relapse.

So with Jeff's help, I cut back on my workouts and increased my food intake slightly. Eventually my weight settled at around 275 pounds. That might seem like a lot, but keep in mind that I am six foot four and a large-framed man. Even at 275, my waist was only 38 inches. I was fit and trim. I looked good and felt better. There was no deprivation. I stopped feeling like I was always on a diet. I didn't have to push myself through punishing workouts.

The excess skin didn't bother me as much at my higher weight. Yes, I still had quite a bit—Jeff guessed between 10 and 15 pounds—but even with the skin, which my clothes hid, no one ever guessed my weight at more than 230 pounds. I carried it well, and I was grateful for that. So I made a conscious decision to drop my disappointment—and the loose skin—at the Lord's feet.

## Occasional Failure Is Part of the Journey

If you are reading this book and thinking that once I settled in at 275 pounds I never had to think about food choices or exercise again, you would be mistaken. For most of us who are struggling to release weight in sin, relapse is common. Whether it comes in the form of a chocolate binge, a shopping spree, a week spent on the couch watching pornography, or a pity party, one slip doesn't have to mean that you're doomed and should stop surrendering your life to God. It's just a sign that a spiritual course correction may be needed.

I have had many, many slips since settling in at my goal weight.

Sharing unhealthy foods with well-meaning friends

Eating to compensate for career setbacks and personal rejection

Making poor food choices while on tour

Finding reasons to avoid working out

Every slip is a signpost on my walk with the Lord. How I choose to respond to the slip determines whether I stay on the main road or end up getting sidetracked. It's an opportunity to practice perseverance. This requires action.

One of the most important actions I take is keeping a food journal. At Jeff's urging, I kept a food journal during much of my weight-loss journey. After I hit my goal weight, I stopped for a while. But whenever I found myself overeating, I returned to writing down my food. I had days when I wanted to do right but didn't. *I keep failing,* I would write. *I thought I was going to do well today, but circumstances got the best of me.*

Keeping a journal helps me in a variety of ways, not all food related.

**It reveals the real issues.** Food is rarely the real issue. Most of my slips are the result of deeply ingrained ways of responding to people and situations in my life. When I'm living inside the Lord's will for me, I am blessed with new ways of responding that don't involve overeating. But if I slack off on any of my spiritual practices, I revert to old patterns of responding. Journaling helps me stay in touch with the real issues so I don't get off track.

**It keeps me honest.** My brain's default setting is a state of amnesia about what goes into my mouth. Anyone who is carrying weight in sin has the same amnesia. *If I don't think about it, maybe I didn't really eat it,* I think. Being committed to rigorous honesty in my journal is the antidote to addictive amnesia.

**It helps me keep momentum.** Having a complete record of my food intake was a useful tool for Jeff, especially as I approached my goal weight. He reviewed my journal on a regular basis and suggested changes in my eating plan. Now if I get off track, I use the journal to see what foods I'm choosing and make the corrections needed to restore momentum.

**It keeps me accountable.** If I have to write it down, I won't eat it. My journal was a college-rule confessional that kept me accountable. This works best if you commit to sharing your journal with a trainer, food coach, or accountability partner.

**It reveals patterns.** I can look back in my journal and connect my slips with what was going on in my life at the time. This makes it easier to find the links between eating and emotions, which gives me the power to choose new responses next time.

**It reveals my progress and gives me hope.** Journaling is a way of documenting the journey. This is an ancient practice. The children of Israel built memorials to remind themselves of the places where they met God. My journal is a memorial to the times I met God through my addictions. It's a testament to how He came through for me. If I'm having an issue, I don't have to worry about it because I can look back and see what I did to deal with a similar issue earlier in my journey. I know that if I do the same things today, I will be fine.

Journaling takes time. There's no way around it. But it's what I need to do in order to keep my occasional slips from becoming so discouraging that they lead to permanent failure.

## Career Perseverance

My weight-loss story isn't the only part of my life where I needed to persevere. My career challenges were even more overwhelming. There were many setbacks. Each had the potential to derail both my future as a musician and the weight loss that held the key to it.

After I settled into a comfortable weight, things just didn't happen fast enough for me. *I'm sure 2005 will be my year to hit it big,* I thought.

It wasn't.

I was making appearances at churches as part of my Training Wills ministry, but there wasn't much interest in my music beyond the pews. When was my big break going to happen? "God, You said to lose weight, and I've done that," I prayed. "How much longer do I have to wait?"

The making of my first record, *Start Somewhere,* is a great example of the power of perseverance in my music career. It's hard to launch any new career, but it's especially brutal in the music business. After many slammed doors, many noes, and many disappointments, I finally rounded up the money to make the album.

During my first day in the studio, everything that could go wrong did. The computer powering the mixing system kept crashing. Was this a sign that I shouldn't be recording this album? Was the Lord trying to tell me to get a day job? The crashes happened so often that I couldn't help but wonder. What did these setbacks really mean?

*You know what they mean,* said the enemy. *They mean that you're a fool for even trying to record this stupid album. Who do you think you are, anyway?*

As I sat with my head in my hands waiting for the recording engineer to reboot the system for the sixth time, a teaching I had heard from James Ryle came to mind. "Prosperity is not coming to a barrier and saying, 'I guess it's not the Lord's will,'" he said. "Prosperity is when you know that God says you can overcome and you can go beyond the barrier, because you know that God said, 'The process is when you prosper.'"

I realized that I could perceive these computer glitches in one of two ways. I could tell myself that they were evidence that recording this album was not the Lord's will for me. Or I could tell myself that these technical difficulties were merely barriers for me to leap over in the process of doing God's will—like hurdles in a track meet.

I chose the latter. *This just might be a season when I need to fight,* I told myself, and I asked the Lord for courage to continue.

Technical problems weren't the only battles I faced during the recording of *Start Somewhere.* My relationship with my trainer had been strained for a while. Something was happening with him, and I wasn't sure what it was. My once encouraging trainer was now cynical, especially about Training Wills, my weight-loss ministry.

"How much longer do you think you can talk about your weight loss?" he kept asking me. "It's old news. Nobody wants to hear about it anymore."

Maybe Jeff was right. Maybe my ministry was past the "sell by" date. But I was still getting invitations to speak. People still wanted to hear my testimony and my music.

As I sat in the studio waiting for the engineers to resolve the last of the technical problems, my phone rang. It was Jeff. He was unhappy about something. I held the phone away from my ear as he yelled. When I ended the call, I knew that our business relationship was over.

I was shaken. How could it be that the person I had looked up to for so long, the man I had trusted so much and relied on so completely, was so lost? It made me question everything. As I tucked my phone into my back pocket, the producer, Sal, told me that he was finally ready to start recording again.

"Oh, Sal, I can't do it," I said, sighing. "I'm just going to go home, because I can't take this."

Sal looked at me. "Are you sure?" he asked. Actually, I wasn't sure. Why did this phone call have to happen right now? Could there be some higher purpose? Could it be just another hurdle in the race? Did the ranting of a man who was clearly having his own problems have to be the reason I walked away from the studio today?

"Wait a minute," I said to Sal. "You know what? I make worship music. People who listen to worship music are often broken, and I am so broken right now."

Could I actually make it through the session without breaking down in sadness over the loss of my friend, my business partner, and my mentor? I wouldn't know unless I tried.

My heart was in my throat. "Sal, hit record," I said. The

music track for "Gonna Make It (After All)" began. When it was time for me to sing, I poured every ounce of anguish, hurt, and betrayal I was feeling into that song and every other track on the album.

The result was something special. Brokenness is embedded in every song on *Start Somewhere*, but nowhere more powerfully than in "Unrestrained." People have told me hundreds of times since that there is something about that song that just grabs them and pulls them in.

Who knew that the horrible ending of a once loving personal and business relationship would be the very thing that the Lord would use to anoint my record? Once again, it proves that I don't know the first thing about how God works.

By trusting God and persevering, I transferred the energy from the obstacles in my path into every song, which created a powerful debut album that opened many doors for me. If I had listened to the voice of the enemy, I would not be writing this book for you now. The Lord is involved in our lives, but we can't always see it. He wants to be a part of everything we do. He wants to join in with us. He wants to be on our side. God was saying, *I know you think this little trial is meant to hurt you, but it's not. I'm about to make you a record that everybody is going to love. I know that Jeff's call kind of messed you up, but if you can get a different perspective about this, you'll realize that it's going to be great.*

If I had stopped right there and said, "Sal, I'm going home," I would have come back a day later, sung my songs, and created a rather ordinary first album. But God wanted this to be extraordinary.

Many of the lessons I've learned on my weight-loss journey came together in the recording studio that day. By trusting

God, keeping my eyes on the vision, and taking up a new perspective, I was blessed with the willingness to persist despite all the obstacles. I cried and screamed and kicked, but I stuck with it, and the results were life changing.

## Count It All Joy

When you're facing barriers like the ones I faced in the recording studio that day, it's easy to think that you're the only one who has to deal with obstacles. Whether the challenges are happening in your career or in your journey to release weight in sin, it's easy to fall prey to the enemy, who wants you to think that you are being singled out for hardship.

That's one of my main motivations for writing this book. If the Lord can help me look at obstacles in a new way and keep me going in spite of them, He can do the same for you. No matter what your weight in sin, you are not alone as you encounter obstacles to your recovery. Your situation is not hopeless.

James 1:2-4 makes it clear how we are to view the obstacles in our lives:

> *Dear brothers and sisters, when troubles come your way, consider it an opportunity for great joy. For you know that when your faith is tested, your endurance has a chance to grow. So let it grow, for when your endurance is fully developed, you will be perfect and complete, needing nothing.*

Be glad, James is saying. The obstacles you dread will produce wonderful results if you let the Lord have His way with you.

Christ is the ultimate example of perseverance. He endured the Cross until the end, but He didn't do it for Himself; He did it for us. He died on the cross, and it looked like His story was over. His mother, disciples, and friends thought it was over. But we know that wasn't the end of the story.

A pastor I know talked about Easter weekend this way: "A lot of us are stuck on Saturday, between the tragedy and Sunday," he said. "We see the tragedy on Friday, but we're on Saturday and we have no idea that Sunday is coming. If people knew that Sunday was going to happen, Friday's tragedy would not seem so scary."

Christ was able to endure the Cross because He knew how the story would end. Can you imagine what was going through His mind? The human part of Him had to be distracted by the incredible physical agony of hanging on the cross after the brutal treatment He had endured. The God part of Him might have been shaking His head, sighing at the hopeless futility of these humans who seem pathologically incapable of seeing the big picture. *When will they get it?* He might have said to Himself. *They only think they're defeating Me. Boy, are they in for a surprise!*

The Lord made the ultimate sacrifice for our salvation, yet He asks so little from us. The only thing He really wants from us is a willingness to look at our obstacles in a different way. He wants us to remember that we have the Creator of the universe on our side. Those obstacles that look like boulders are really only pebbles. They are not to be feared. Lean into them with confidence.

How will you respond to the barriers you encounter during your journey?

# CHAPTER 11

# ARE YOU COMMITTED OR JUST INTERESTED?

WHAT DOES IT REALLY MEAN when we make a New Year's resolution to . . .

> lose weight
>
> work out at the gym
>
> quit smoking
>
> quit drinking
>
> give up the porn

. . . and then throw in the towel by the middle of February?

We've all done it. I've done it. I have made the diet resolution on New Year's Eve and broken it by noon on New Year's Day—not just once but dozens of times.

What does it really mean?

It means that I wasn't really committed. If I had been, I would have kept those resolutions.

The truth is, I wasn't committed at all. I was just interested.

Is it the same for you? Let's say that you have a spending problem and want to get out of debt.

You are *interested* if you buy a book on living within your means, read the first few chapters, abandon the book to your nightstand, and don't change your spending habits at all.

You are *committed* if you complete a Dave Ramsey financial course, follow his principles, pay off all your bills, and start living debt free.

Let's say that you are overweight and want to get in shape.

You are *interested* if you buy a gym membership, go once, and then find every excuse in the book not to go.

You are *committed* if you work with a trainer for a year and end up losing 200 pounds.

You may believe that you are committed when you make the promise to start the diet tomorrow or to quit smoking in the New Year or to join the gym on Monday. "This time I'm really serious," you announce to anyone who will listen. But in reality you are just interested.

The difference between being committed and being interested is action. When you're interested, you gather information, talk about it, and think about it. But beyond the idea rolling around in your brain and your lips moving when you talk about it, there's little action.

Committed people translate their intentions into concrete actions.

What made me committed instead of just interested was the fact that I had promised my trainer that I would stick with it for ninety days. Deep down, I wanted to find an excuse to be fat forever. Part of me wanted to fail so I could say to the Lord, "See, I told You this wasn't going to work."

I was actually mad at God after making my ninety-day commitment to Jeff. My thoughts veered from the negative and sarcastic . . . *Okay, if this is supposed to work, Lord, I'm kind of mad at You. I'm fighting with You. You're making me change, and I don't like it!* . . . to weary resignation . . . *Okay, Lord* (sigh), *I'm going to do it. You put Jeff in my path, and he said to give it a try for just ninety days. Okay* (sigh). *This is what I'm going to do. I'm going to try it. I'm going to play by the rules.* . . . to defiance . . . *But if it doesn't work, I'm not going to keep this up. I'm not going to live my life going back and forth.*

I was committed to doing my part, but I knew that my strength alone wouldn't be enough. My own strength had gotten me to the point of morbid obesity! So I prayed, *Lord, if I'm going to do my part, then You have to help.*

And as you already know, I started the ninety-day process committed but impatient. For the first thirty days, I was obsessed with my body, desperate for evidence that I was getting smaller. As the days crept by, it didn't seem like anything was changing. I was frustrated.

And then, by the ninety-day point, the tiny changes that had happened to my body each day had added up. I didn't notice them, and the people I saw frequently didn't notice them. But the people I hadn't seen in three months did. I felt like I had received a medal of honor that said, "This is working!" I was now committed and inspired instead of committed and impatient.

Today I see the significance of the ninety-day commitment, and I have noticed three-month cycles everywhere. Buy furniture and get ninety days same as cash. Seasons are ninety days long. People in twelve-step programs start sponsoring others after ninety days of sobriety.

There is great wisdom in making short-term commitments to change and renewing those commitments on a regular basis. Eventually those short-term commitments accumulate to create long-term change.

For the next ninety days, what will you be? Committed or just interested?

CHAPTER **12**

# BEWARE OF COMPLACENCY

ON MY WEIGHT-LOSS JOURNEY, encouragement from others helped me persevere. Friends noticed my shrinking size and urged me on. When I reached my goal, everyone cheered. But then something happened. As the months wore on, people who had been my biggest supporters seemed to develop a case of amnesia. Every once in a while friends would pull out pictures from my past and say with amazement, "I completely forgot that you were that big."

As I met new people in my travels, they met a slim Calvin. They had never seen me fat. This new, normal-size Calvin was the only Calvin they had ever known.

No one was cheering for me anymore. And honestly, I missed the attention.

Maybe it will be the same for you. After the fuss dies down and the praise ends, what will keep you going? How will you stay motivated to live your life without your weight in sin after you've reached your goal?

## Complacent to the Core

Complacency has always been an issue for me. When I was young, I often thought about giving weight loss a try. But then I thought about all the obstacles. What would I do if it was too hard? If I thought there was any chance of failure, I'd give up before I even started. Even though God was saying, *Calvin, I'll bless whatever you put your hand to,* I wouldn't put my hand to anything because I was afraid I might fail. I talked myself out of trying before I even started because the obstacles seemed insurmountable. The what-ifs were paralyzing. Eating doughnuts seemed to help.

During my weight-loss journey, complacency receded into the background as I learned how to focus on God's vision for me and take up a new perspective. It was exciting. For the first time ever, I realized that if I handed the problem over to the Lord and let go of my old ideas, I could accomplish what seemed impossible. As a result, the Lord blessed my weight loss supernaturally. You couldn't get me to eat a doughnut. You could dangle one in front of my mouth or pass a box right under my nose, and it wouldn't break my resolve.

After maintaining my weight for a few months, I looked back at my old pictures. I was astounded and humbled. I knew that I was a living, breathing, walking miracle. I was still focused, still energized, and still eager to live this new way of life. I was proud of what I had accomplished, yet very aware that it had come through the grace of God alone. My testimony was inspiring people to confess their weight in sin and make real changes in their lives. In the process, people were hearing and loving my music, just as God had promised. Doughnuts had lost their appeal.

As time passed, however, I grew more accustomed to living life in a normal-size body. I was still focused on my original vision, but there were other things to think about—like my music career. After all, God had told me to lose the weight first and then I could take the story of my victory through Him to the world—along with my songs.

I took the Lord's directive seriously. If the Creator speaks, the created listen, right? I threw myself into my career, going out on the road for weeks on end. The constant travel took me out of my comfort zone and thrust me into a strange new world where the only routine was the fact that there was no routine.

On the road, I had no control over my environment. Unable to afford an entourage to recreate the conditions that had supported my weight loss at home, I found it hard to stick to a workout schedule. Hotel gyms were inadequate. There was no trainer around to motivate me.

Each time I left home to tour, I promised myself that I would work out and eat right. In a matter of days, however, something would happen. A well-meaning host would put a plate of delicious food in front of my face. How could I say no without seeming ungrateful? I would pick up the fork and dig in.

Every time I arrived back home in Nashville after weeks away, my apartment was dark and quiet. But my heart was even darker. Despite my best intentions, despite my promises that this time would be different, I would return home sick with the realization that yet again I had eaten too much, exercised too little, and fallen prey to fears I thought I had surrendered to God long ago. I would sit in the dark at my kitchen table wondering if the sacrifices were worth the blessings yet to come— blessings like a hit song, a woman to share my life with, and financial security. It seemed like some of the blessings I had already received were slipping away, like comfort in my body and confidence in my ability to make good choices.

There were also new fears.

My weight was inching upward. I could feel it in my clothes and see it in the mirror. Terror engulfed me. My entire livelihood was built on a story of victory over my weight in sin, and there I was, taking it back the same way I had taken it off. I was picking up small change—one pizza slice, one BBQ rib, one spoonful of ice cream at a time. Doughnuts were starting to look appealing again.

Pressure to stay thin mounted, as did the reasons to eat. I was developing new business relationships all over the country, and doors to new opportunities were opening every day. Unfortunately I didn't have any staff to handle things for me, and there simply weren't enough hours in the day to get things done. In addition, since I was a new recording artist, some radio stations didn't want to play my music. The rejection devastated me, and I resorted to old coping strategies. Doughnuts helped.

As demand for my music grew, interest in my weight-loss ministry shrank. Jeff's words echoed in my head: "Your story will get old, and no one will want to hear it." In my heart of hearts, I was afraid he might be right.

The clear vision of my future that had once burned so brightly in my mind now flickered like a tiny television in the next room.

Eating seemed like a good way to ease the pain. Just one bite wouldn't hurt. By now I had forgotten an essential truth about my relationship with food. If I'm eating outside my boundaries, "just one" always leads to the whole box.

I knew what to do, but I couldn't bring myself to do it. I had all the tools, but I refused to pick them up. Old character issues like pride and fear were back with a vengeance. I knew that if I didn't get back on track, my story of victory would quickly become a source of embarrassment. I was self-conscious. The enemy was jubilant.

When people looked at me, what were they thinking? Were they judging me? I never knew for sure. As my clothes got tighter, I considered my options.

Bulimia? Too messy. I hated to throw up.

Anorexia? Not possible. I liked to eat too much.

Gastric bypass surgery? I was no longer fat enough to qualify. Oh, the irony!

During the days I spent at home between road trips, I still believed I could get the magic back simply by returning to my old eating and exercising routines. But nothing was the same anymore. My new trainer always seemed to be unavailable just when I got back into town. Without that encouragement, I sank deeper into old habits. All the external forces I had come to rely on seemed out of reach.

Why couldn't I get it back?

## When Do I Graduate?

I wish I could tell you that once you've lost your weight in sin—whatever it is—life can go back to normal.

Unfortunately, it just doesn't work that way.

Unless the behavior changes you made on the way to your goal become integrated into the way you live after you reach your goal, old habits will inevitably return. They did for me.

After perseverance comes vigilance.

If you want to stay in shape, you will always have to work

out, especially as you get older. This fundamental rule of physics applies to even naturally thin professional athletes. If you stop working out and let age take its course, you will eventually get weak and flabby. God doesn't reward your hard work by granting you a permanent exemption from these basic laws of nature. People who lose a lot of weight don't automatically get a highly stoked metabolism that allows them to eat whatever they want.

It's the same for every lifestyle change.

Anyone who overcomes weight in sin must do two things to keep from backsliding:

Continue to abstain from the destructive behavior.

Maintain a spiritual exercise program that keeps compulsions at bay.

Here's where it gets challenging. When we release our weight in sin, life becomes full and interesting—so much so that the spiritual habits we developed during our journey are often the first things to go when we get too busy.

The very things I had once done so enthusiastically to stay on track during my journey became unwelcome obligations at the bottom of my daily to-do list. Eating right and exercising became second-tier priorities. My relationship with the Lord— the thing that had made my successful journey possible in the first place—sank to the very bottom.

As my schedule got busier, I found it tough to set aside time for prayer and the Word. There were so many other things to do. And besides, I was already very spiritual. I knew the Bible inside and out. People looked up to me as a leader, a towering spiritual presence with a voice so big that it brought people sobbing to the altar. I was obviously anointed.

My mobile GPS unit summed up my spiritual prowess

better than anything else: "You have arrived," cooed the synthetic female voice. I loved hearing that phrase.

And then one day I stepped on the scale and recoiled in horror. I had picked up change to the tune of 30 extra pounds.

I had arrived—at a roadside rest stop on the return trip to obesity.

## The Way Out

My story isn't unique. It's actually older than old. You'll find this same story line in many great tales in the Bible.

1. Life gets bad.
2. Man finds God.
3. Life gets better.
4. Man forgets God.
5. Repeat steps 1–4.

My complacency had morphed into an arrogant self-reliance that set me above others and told me I no longer needed God. I wasn't spending time in prayer. I wasn't reading Scripture. My relationship with the Lord was no longer the priority in my life.

God doesn't often work in the hearts of people who secretly believe that they don't need Him. He respectfully allowed me to step out of His will and try it my way for a while. And in the process, those towering spiritual gifts—my voice and my story—were quickly becoming liabilities. Left to my own devices, I would soon be known as that fat singer who built his career on a weight-loss story and ended up having to be cut out of his home by firemen with chain saws.

My story is a great illustration of a spiritual principle that I had to learn the hard way:

*Any strength overused becomes a weakness.*

Because I was convinced that I had the spiritual thing mastered, I ended up closing myself off from the very power that had healed me.

A pastor I know put it this way: "God will never take you to a point where you can regard Him as useless," he said. Ironically, the more success I had, the more I thought I could do it on my own. The better the results, the more I believed that my past success had occurred because of me and any future success depended totally upon me. Gradually, I factored God right out of the equation as I dreamed about the praise I would get from adoring fans in the future. (I wanted to have fans so rabid that I would have to hire someone just to handle the restraining orders.)

When I stopped to look at where I was going, it occurred to me that the rock stardom I had in mind was very different from the life of someone who had once been my hero: Jesus Christ. The original reluctant rock star, Christ was hounded by friends, followers, and enemies in much the same way that celebrities are stalked by fans and the paparazzi today.

But Christ wasn't concerned about self-promotion. He wasn't surrounded by handlers, bodyguards, press agents, and hairstylists. No one was there to separate the brown M&M's from the rest of the colors. Christ had a job to do, and He was all business. He had humanity to save.

After Christ performed miracles, He wasn't thinking about whether cameras were there to record the anomaly. He was always thinking about where He had to be next. He never rested on His laurels by focusing on how good His last miracle was.

In fact, He rarely talked about His miracles, and He certainly never bragged. I doubt that Christ ever said, "Boy, I really out-did Myself yesterday when I raised Lazarus from the dead." His words probably sounded more like this: "I've got to get over to Bethlehem next, and by the way, don't tell anybody about what I did for you today."

Christ knew that His vision, His purpose, His goal was the Cross. His eyes never wavered.

But mine did. I took my eyes off the process.

## Coasting Is Costly

The enemy says, *Relax. You have an early flight. You can put off your morning prayers until you're on the plane.* He is a master of subtlety, suggesting that we can delay or avoid the things we need to do.

*God will understand,* the enemy continues. *You've been work-ing so hard. You can coast for a while.* The enemy is persistent, but he leaves out an important fact. We can only coast in one direction: downhill.

Every skipped prayer, every blown-off Bible study, every missed morning meditation, every half-finished gratitude list represents a chink in my spiritual armor. The enemy squeals in delight every time I make a choice that proves that my relation-ship with God is not my first priority.

The enemy knows that whatever I value more than God I will lose. And that's the enemy's goal. He wants me to lose it all and wallow in despair.

Honestly, I was putting a lot before God—my tour, my next album, and my ministry, just for starters. Everything I had worked for was at risk because I had forgotten that being healed from weight in sin is an inside job that is never finished. There is no graduation date. Without realizing it, I had turned my focus outward in my search for relief. If circumstances would just line up the way I wanted them to, then I could get back on track. If only I could find the right trainer, travel less, find a new gym, or get my stomach stapled, then things would be okay.

God was counting on me to keep putting Him first, and I had failed. He had all sorts of encouragement ready for me, but I was too busy to listen. God knew that my career would take off when I lost the weight. He knew that the pressure would increase, and the demands on my time would grow. *Just stay with Me,* God might have said to me when I brought my workout scheduling problems to Him in prayer. *I'll show you how to get it all done.* He had so many exciting new experiences in store for me. Some would feel good and some would feel bad, but He was counting on me to come to Him for the lowdown on what it all meant: *You can't see the big picture, but I can.* If I had poured out my pain about my setbacks, He was waiting to tell me, *There really is nothing to fear.* If I had come to Him in tears about a broken business relationship, He might have said, *You have no idea what blessing awaits you just around the corner.* If I had explained my fear about saying no to people who wanted to feed me unhealthy foods, He would have had a complete library of responses ready for me: *You don't have to worry about what others think, because I'll be giving you the words to say.*

While the Lord was waiting patiently for me to drop my bag of troubles at His feet, I was being distracted by a laughing snake dressed as an airport skycap who told me that he would carry the bag for me. Guess who was left holding the bag?

## From Rebellion to Reliance

After months of struggles, one thing was clear. My 30-pound weight gain wasn't a food problem. It wasn't an exercise problem. It was a God problem. I had stepped back into the role of manager of my own life, and I had failed.

More than anything, I wanted to feel the freedom that I sing about in "Unrestrained."

I was defeated, and God knew it. I was done trying to do things my way. Fortunately, freedom was only a prayer away: *Lord, help me to put You first and to see my life the way You see it.*

How did the Lord get me back on track?

> **He reminded me to put Him first.** I once again got my marching orders from the Lord by spending time in prayer. No longer did I try to shoehorn my prayers in between "more important" things or relegate time with the Lord to the end of the day when my energy was flagging. God got the best of me, not the leftovers.

> **He asked me to tell my story.** The Lord moved me to step up my efforts to help others. This was a surprise. As I struggled with the return to old habits, I had stopped sharing my story because I felt defeated. God had other ideas for me. *Share it. Share all of it,* He said. *If you want to keep the gifts I give you, you must give them away.* So I did. Little did I know how powerfully my story would move others who had released their weight in sin and then taken it back again.

> **He taught me to depend on Him, not people.** The Lord revealed to me that I tend to rely too much on people and not enough on Him. My utter dependence on a

trainer for motivation and accountability was a prime example. When my trainer was gone, I wouldn't work out. Today I turn to God for motivation. Though the enemy still taunts me for my childlike reliance on God, I know that He is the only source of true power.

**He helped me set realistic expectations.** It is still hard to eat right and work out when I'm traveling. But I realized I was setting myself up for failure by expecting that I could come home from a tour weighing less than when I left. Today my goal is to maintain my weight when I'm on the road—not gain or lose. If the travel becomes too overwhelming and I think I'm going to fall back into old patterns, I take time off to recharge.

**He showed me His big picture.** After I lost weight, I focused on just one aspect of God's vision for me (the music), but I did so at the expense of the thorn— my weight in sin—that had led me to depend on God in the first place. The longer it took for my singing career to take off, the more discouraged I became and the less I was able to focus on God's complete vision for my life. I was out of balance. Reconnecting with God's vision helped me restore that balance.

**He made me accountable to others.** As my complacency grew, I lost touch with accountability partners and friends who knew the real me. I stopped connecting with people who would shine the light on my blind spots and call me on my behavior quirks and attitude problems. God has given me a new willingness to listen to people I trust and accept their feedback, even if it is uncomfortable.

## A Season of Integrity

I can now see how God lovingly let me wander off until the consequences of complacency drove me back into His arms. He showed me all the ways I still withheld parts of my life from Him and how eager I was to take back control over others. He showed me that my physical size isn't the only barometer of fitness. I have been obese and defiant, and I have been slim and defiant. Either way, my quality of life deteriorates quickly when I think I'm running the show.

Above all, this phase of my journey has driven home the importance of spiritual fitness. I'm working with the ultimate trainer—God—whose regimen is producing a resilient, resourceful, and reliant Calvin who is able to handle both triumphs and setbacks with uncommon grace. With God's help, I am focusing more on the inward man while continuing to care for the outer man by eating right and working out. As a result, God is changing me from the inside out. He is reprogramming my heart and my mind, transforming the way I view myself and others. He is rightsizing me in every possible way: physically, emotionally, and spiritually. For that, I am eternally grateful.

How will you use the lessons of complacency to deepen your reliance on the Lord?

CHAPTER **13**

# FROM MISERY TO MOTIVATION

WHEN I THINK BACK over my life, I am amazed. I knew that the Lord was a big God, but I had no idea just how big until I made the decision to surrender my weight in sin to Him. God is big enough to heal even Big Cal.

God used my biggest source of shame—a body so large that everyone around me knew the truth I was desperately trying to hide—and turned it into the biggest blessing of my life. The little boy once known as "rock head" has even been called a Christian rock star on occasion.

The Lord transformed my misery into ministry. He took the elements of my character that were driving my desire to over-eat—my pride, my fears, my insecurities, my way of looking at the world—and converted them into a powerful force that has been a catalyst for His healing power to change many lives.

God also turned my misery into motivation, and He can do the same for you. He will take your secret sin from you if you let Him. He wants to take you from bondage to freedom. If you are completely bankrupt and simply don't have the energy to try it your way anymore, you are just one tiny prayer away from the beginning of your journey.

*Lord, I can't carry this anymore. You can.*

Can you hear the ground shudder and see the puff of dust rising when you drop your weight in sin at the Lord's feet? Can you feel your spirits lift as you realize that you no longer have to try to figure this out on your own?

It can happen for you.


**Eight Steps to Freedom**

This book is the story of an ordinary man's weight loss. But it isn't a diet book. It isn't an exercise book. It's not a book for anyone who wants to look like a bodybuilder. It's a book for the everyday person who is tired of the quick-fix promises, the schemes, and the failures. It's for the person who is ready to throw in the towel and look for a different kind of fitness—spiritual fitness—brought about by God-inspired workouts that produce lasting results and offer the best guarantee against relapse.

You've seen how this spiritual fitness program works in eight simple steps:

1. Own your own weight.
2. See God as your friend.
3. Take up a new perspective.
4. Get someone to hold you accountable.
5. Start somewhere.
6. Eliminate the excuses.
7. Accept the need for training wheels.
8. Persevere to the end.

These steps transformed my life and continue to do so today. They can do the same for you. They will open the door for God to enter your heart, mind, and soul and dismantle the thought patterns and beliefs that drive your compulsions.

This spiritual fitness program will break you, and then it will heal you. Instead of living a life filled with drama, obsession, and angst, you will find yourself becoming a living and breathing example of triumph over adversity.

God created us to be solutions in life, not problems. He wants to use your experience to show others what can be true in their lives. God believes in the power of example. Why shouldn't that example be you?

If you are still being held hostage by the enemy, who tells you that your secret weight in sin is too much for even God to handle, I offer my story as evidence to the contrary. It is possible to live a life free and unrestrained.

## God Lifts Every Weight

Without fail, every time I give my testimony, at least one person comes up to me afterward and tells me about his or her hidden weight. Dozens have come clean about their secret shame, confessing their slavery to drugs, homosexuality, pornography, and more. They tell me that the physical transformation they see in me gives them hope that the Lord can do for them what He has done for me: take misery and turn it into ministry.

The thing that held me back for so long—my weight—is the very thing that God is using to help others. Their stories are striking. Here are just a few.

**Honor thy parents.** A slim, rough-around-the-edges white man in his fifties approached me one day after I had shared my testimony at a church service. His raspy voice said "smoker." His weathered hands said "laborer." His rough skin said "I probably have little in common with you."

But his eyes said something else. "I just wanted to tell you that your testimony really blessed me," Steve whispered, reaching out and clasping my hands as his eyes welled with tears. "I got into my car after I heard your testimony, and I picked up change."

My heart swelled with gratitude, and I offered up a silent prayer of praise. I thought that like me, maybe Steve had fought the battle of the bulge and with God's help had won.

What Steve said next surprised me, however. "Yeah, I got in the car, picked up the phone, and called my mother for the first time in twenty years. I haven't seen her in thirty." He paused to wipe a tear from his face. "After hearing you talk about picking up change, I started looking for the weight in my own life. And there it was—the weight I had been carrying for so long. I realized that I couldn't carry the weight of shutting her out of my life any longer."

My weight-loss testimony had motivated a skinny man to call his mother. And after doing so, he looked like the weight of the world had been lifted from his shoulders.

That's when it hit me. My testimony wasn't about weight. It was about burdens. It was about the heaviness we carry because of the relationships we have with ourselves, with others, with things, and with our past. Everyone is carrying something.

**Falsely accused.** "Can I just talk to you?" a man with a sad face and glazed eyes asked after I had shared my testimony.

"I'm a teacher. I have been falsely accused of sexual molestation," whispered this man we'll call Joe. "This is the first time I've been able to cry. I felt like if I cried, I was giving in to the accusation. When I heard you sing the song 'Receive,' I just let it all out. I have held it in for so long, and I just wanted to thank you."

It was clear to me that he needed a release—someone he could talk to who wouldn't judge him. He just wanted to feel loved.

In "Receive," I sing about receiving God's love, which may have been especially meaningful to Joe because he didn't feel like he was loved at all. His story was in the news, and he couldn't find another job to save his life. I don't know what happened to Joe after that; I pray that he was able to lay aside his weight and move on.

**Sexual shame.** Not long ago I was singing "Receive" and talking about how much God loves us. Though the audience was filled with people who weren't overweight, they were responding to my song in visible ways. One man approached me after the service and broke down. He had been molested by his uncle as a boy and it was weighing heavy on him.

As I listened to his story, I could see the guilt, shame, and remorse he was carrying. I knew that it was hard for him to believe that God can love us so much despite our shortcomings. But He can. He does.

## Give the Weight to God

There is hope. The main message in my ministry is this: God specializes in taking the pain. In fact, He has been anxiously waiting for this moment. He has been waiting for you to realize that your weight is too big for you to carry on your own.

The key is letting Him do it. Like a small child with a broken toy, we need to take our problem to Daddy and let Him fix it. We must be completely willing to drop our weight, whatever it is, and let God pick it up and work on it.

Starting somewhere—picking up change—means being willing to let go. If we have even the smallest inkling that we can do this by ourselves, the Lord won't take the burden. He'll wait patiently while we continue to try to handle it ourselves.

But the moment we surrender the weight, all His power suddenly becomes available to us. And it's a lot of power. After all, we're dealing with the Creator of the universe here. No matter what our weight is, no matter how heavy it is, no matter how hopeless it seems or how long we've been carrying it, God is big enough to handle the job.

Think about it. Jesus hung out with sinners. Talk about a rough crowd! The apostle Paul started out as a virtual serial killer. These people were checking extra bags at Satan International Airport. But that didn't stop Jesus from caring about them. Unlike us, He wasn't focusing on what they were; He was focused on what they could be. He could see their potential. And ultimately, their weight in sin was the gateway to a life that none of them could have imagined. That ragtag band of losers ended up changing the world. In fact, because of them, the Lord's message of hope reached you and me!

You have the same potential. You can have a life free from slavery to behaviors you can't stop, thoughts you can't silence, and appetites you can't satisfy.

Starting somewhere means being willing to let go of your weight in sin and start the journey.

Are you ready?

# The Ways and Means of Losing 215 Pounds

How does an ordinary person lose 215 pounds without medical intervention?

Trust God.

Eat less.

Move more.

Understand that there are no quick fixes.

Traditional diet and exercise books tell you what to eat and how to move. Millions of pages are devoted to describing sample meal plans and workouts that few can stick to for long. If you're lucky, a typical diet book may dedicate a page or two to the emotional or spiritual reasons behind overeating.

This book takes the opposite approach. Thirteen chapters are devoted to the God part of the solution. This short appendix is dedicated to diet and exercise.

I decided to include it because people always want to know how I did it. This section answers those questions. Excerpts from my food journals give you a glimpse of what I ate during the early days of my weight-loss journey. Simple workouts designed by Dino Nowak, my current trainer, will help you start somewhere, no matter what shape you are in today.

As you read this section, please remember two things. First, check with your doctor before starting any diet or exercise program. Second, if you try to follow my eating and exercise plan without truly surrendering to the Lord, this will be just another failed weight-loss attempt.

The Lord wants a lot more than that for you.

## Sample Meal Plans

I rarely cook. Most of my meals are made out of a box or eaten in restaurants. This sample fourteen-day menu, taken directly from my own food journal, gives you plenty of brand-name food choices that you can mix and match. It is possible to eat healthy on the go!

| DAY | BREAKFAST | LUNCH | DINNER | SNACK |
|---|---|---|---|---|
| 1 | three egg whites and one whole egg with vegetables and grilled chicken; one slice of multigrain bread | turkey on sun-dried tomato wrap with lettuce, tomato, pickle, and onion; side of cottage cheese with honey mustard from Jersey Mike's | MangoFest smoothie from Smoothie King (35 ounces) | |

| DAY | BREAKFAST | LUNCH | DINNER | SNACK |
|---|---|---|---|---|
| 2 | instant oatmeal (maple and brown sugar); egg substitute on homemade wheat tortilla | Healthy Choice meal of fish, rice, and vegetables; one pear | chicken and vegetable stir-fry with teriyaki sauce | Kashi bar (honey and almond flax); low-fat organic strawberry yogurt |
| 3 | three egg whites and one whole egg with vegetables and grilled chicken; one slice of multigrain bread from Coffee Beanery | turkey on sun-dried tomato wrap with lettuce, tomato, pickle, and onion; side of cottage cheese with honey mustard | MangoFest smoothie from Smoothie King (35 ounces) | Kashi bar; watermelon; grapes |
| 4 | bowl of oatmeal from Cracker Barrel with one scoop of brown sugar and fifteen raisins; egg substitute on wheat toast, grilled | turkey on sun-dried tomato wrap with lettuce, tomato, pickle, and onion; side of cottage cheese with honey mustard | Lean Cuisine meal: salmon, whole wheat pasta, and spinach in basil sauce | Kashi bar |
| 5 | broiled lemon pepper fish, asparagus, and red potatoes from Wild Oats | turkey on sun-dried tomato wrap with lettuce, tomato, pickle, and onion; side of cottage cheese with honey mustard | MangoFest smoothie from Smoothie King (35 ounces) | Kashi bar |
| 6 | instant oatmeal (maple and brown sugar); three egg whites and one whole egg on whole wheat tortilla | two small Cajun fish fillets (7.6 ounces); vegetable medley (broccoli and carrots); ¼ cup of brown rice | chicken and vegetable stir-fry | Kashi bar; low-fat yogurt |

| DAY | BREAKFAST | LUNCH | DINNER | SNACK |
|---|---|---|---|---|
| 7 | one bowl of oatmeal; one egg; half slice of whole wheat toast | one jerk chicken wrap; grilled asparagus with salt, pepper, and light butter from Saffire | medium 32-ounce smoothie from Smoothie King | three slices of deli turkey; twenty-five grapes |
| 8 | three egg whites and one whole egg with vegetables on stone-ground whole wheat tortilla | turkey on sun-dried tomato wrap with lettuce, tomato, pickle, and onion; side of cottage cheese with honey mustard | chicken and vegetable stir-fry in teriyaki sauce | Kashi bar |
| 9 | three egg whites and one whole egg with vegetables and salsa; one slice of whole wheat toast | Healthy Choice meal: chicken, potatoes, broccoli, and peach dessert | chicken and vegetable stir-fry in teriyaki sauce | Kashi bar; grapes |
| 10 | three egg whites and one whole egg with vegetables and salsa; one slice of whole wheat toast | Healthy Choice meal: salmon and whole wheat pasta | large bowl of minestrone soup | Kashi bar; fruit; Smoothie King smoothie |
| 11 | three egg whites and one whole egg with vegetables and salsa; one slice of whole wheat toast | chicken stir-fry with brown rice | turkey wrap with lettuce, tomato, pickle, and light honey mustard from Subway | Kashi bar |
| 12 | three egg whites and one whole egg with vegetables and salsa; one slice of whole wheat toast | turkey Reuben with Swiss cheese from Jason's Deli; steamed broccoli | salmon; chicken; salad; two scoops of mashed potatoes; asparagus; multigrain bread; fruit | Kashi bar; peanut butter and jelly on thick bread |

| DAY | BREAKFAST | LUNCH | DINNER | SNACK |
|-----|-----------|-------|--------|-------|
| 13 | salmon and asparagus | turkey sub with cheese, mayo, and mustard from Jersey Mike's | lentil soup and chicken Caesar with fat-free feta cheese from Macaroni Grill | Kashi bar |
| 14 | South Beach peanut butter bar | vegetable soup; jerk-grilled chicken wrap with honey mustard, and asparagus from Saffire | teriyaki-glazed salmon on salad from Wolfgang Puck | Kashi bar |

## Sample Workouts

These sample workouts were developed by Dino Nowak, a certified health and weight-loss coach (ACSM, Cooper Institute, ACE).[1] They are very similar to the workouts I used during the early days of my weight-loss journey. Like me, Dino believes that true transformation happens from the inside out and that the emotional and spiritual components of fitness are as important as the physical.

### Tips to Stay on Track

- Exercise in the morning, since this increases the likelihood of sticking with the program. Too often after a long, stressful day, exercise is put off until tomorrow and the downward spiral continues.
- Strive for progress, not perfection. Remember, baseball players are considered successful with a .300 batting average. That means they are successful

---

[1] For more information about Dino Nowak, visit http://www.dinonowak.com.

only three out of ten times. Extend some grace to
yourself and press on.
- Do what you can and log your progress, increasing
  little by little.
- Focus on how you're feeling, the powerful example
  you're setting for your loved ones, and the years you
  are adding to your life. The external results *will* come.
- Remember that victory doesn't come in a standard
  shape or size, so fight to win and don't surrender!

### Sample Seven-Day Program

Be sure to consult with your physician before beginning any
exercise regimen.

You should never have pain in your joints during any of these
movements. If you do experience pain, stop immediately; don't
try to push through it. Move on to something that doesn't hurt.

Before attempting these exercises, see the next section,
"Exercise Descriptions," for more detailed instructions.

#### MONDAY

Chair/couch sit-down, stand-ups with overhead
alternating shoulder press: fifteen to twenty
repetitions

Step-ups on single stair: ten to fifteen repetitions

Stair walks, single step: three to ten times up and down
the staircase

Jogging in place: thirty seconds to one minute of jogging,
then a thirty-second rest; repeat three to five times

Walking with speed intervals: twenty to thirty minutes

**TUESDAY**

Push-ups off countertop: fifteen to twenty repetitions

Laundry detergent or milk jug row: fifteen to twenty repetitions

Arm curl raises with cans: fifteen to twenty repetitions

Imaginary jump rope: thirty seconds to one minute, then rest thirty seconds; repeat three to five times

Walking with speed intervals: twenty to thirty minutes

**WEDNESDAY**

Wall squats: thirty seconds to one minute, then rest one minute; repeat two to three times

Calf raises on stair: fifteen to twenty repetitions

Stair walks, skip a step: three to ten times up and down the staircase (always take single steps on the way down and hold on to the railing)

Jab, jab, punch: twenty per side, then finish with thirty-second flurry

Walking with speed intervals: twenty to thirty minutes

**THURSDAY**

Forty-five- to sixty-minute walk, bike, or swim

**FRIDAY**

Push-ups off countertop: fifteen to twenty reps

Laundry detergent or milk jug row: fifteen to twenty reps

Arm curl raises with cans: fifteen to twenty reps

Combine thirty seconds of each of the following back-to-back, increasing the time for each exercise as you can:

Thirty seconds jogging in place

Thirty seconds imaginary jump rope

Thirty seconds jab, jab, punch on each side

Walking with speed intervals: twenty to thirty minutes

### SATURDAY

Forty-five- to sixty-minute walk, bike, or swim

### SUNDAY

Rest

## Exercise Descriptions

**Arm curl raises:** Stand upright with a soup can or water bottle in each hand. Perform an arm curl, palms up, toward your chest, keeping your elbows tucked into your sides. Lower your arms and then raise them to the side, with palms facing the floor so you form a T. Lower your arms and repeat.

**Calf raises on step:** Stand with both feet on a stair and hold on to a railing or wall. Slide your heels back so they are hanging off the stair. Rise up to your tiptoes, hold two seconds, and then let your heels drop down. Return to the starting position and repeat.

**Chair/couch sit-down, stand-ups with alternating shoulder press:** Start in a seated position on a couch or chair with your feet about hip-width apart. Hold a soup can or water bottle in each hand. Stand up, keeping your heels in contact with the floor at all times. As you stand, press your right arm up to the ceiling, lower it, and then raise and lower your left arm. Return to the seated position and repeat.

**Imaginary jump rope:** Imagine you have a jump rope in your hands and begin to jump rope. Start with small movements, and as you can, jump a little higher and faster. Have fun and try some side-to-side movements, high knees, or other variations.

**Jab, jab, punch:** Stand with your left foot in front and right foot in back. Raise your left arm up into guard position and your right arm back, ready to punch. Perform two quick jabs with your left arm, then punch and follow through with your right arm as you rotate your torso to put some power behind the punch. Repeat the specified number of times, then switch your stance to punch with your left arm, and begin again. At the very end, finish the exercise with a flurry of alternating left and right punches as quickly as you can.

**Jogging in place:** Jog in place, starting with small movements, and as you can, lift your knees higher and run faster.

**Laundry detergent or milk jug row:** If you don't have weights, grab a laundry detergent bottle or milk jug.

Place your left hand on a countertop or the back of a sturdy chair to brace yourself and hold the weight with your right hand. Take a step back with your right leg so the left is in front, then bend from your torso and pull the weight up as if you were starting a lawn mower. Do not round your back. Repeat and then switch sides.

**Push-ups off countertop:** Place your hands on a countertop and position your feet far enough back so that when you come down, the middle of your chest is right above the countertop. Maintain a straight back; don't allow your hips to drop or your backside to stick out. If this is too difficult, just go halfway down. As you become stronger, move to the floor and do a push-up on your knees, working toward a full push-up on your toes.

**Stair walks, single step:** Walk up your stairs one step at a time and then walk back down.

**Stair walks, skip a step:** Walk up your stairs, skipping one step each time while going up if possible. If the steps are too deep, you may not be able to. Always take one step at a time on the way down and hold on to the railing.

**Step-ups on single stair:** Place your right foot on a stair and hold on to a wall or railing for balance. Step your left foot up onto the same stair. Lower and repeat, then switch feet.

**Walking with speed intervals:** Walk around the block, the mall, or anywhere. Every few minutes, increase your walking pace for one minute, then slow it back down for a minute or two until you are ready for another speed interval.

**Wall squats:** Stand with your back against a sturdy wall and place your feet about one and a half feet in front of you. Slide down the wall as if you were sitting in a chair and hold. To make it easier, slide down only a little bit; to make it harder, come down lower. (Your heels should be in contact with the floor at all times, and about 80 percent of your weight should be on your heels. There should be no knee pain at all. If you experience pain, readjust your feet to increase the angle in your knees and do not slide down so far. If you still experience pain, stop and move on to another exercise.)

# Your Turn to Start Somewhere

ONE OF THE THINGS that helped me most in choosing a healthier lifestyle was keeping track of my eating and exercise habits. It was a great way to keep me honest, motivated, and accountable. For that reason, I strongly encourage you to keep a journal of your own. Even if you don't meet your goals for the day, don't get discouraged. Just keep writing down your progress, consider what caused you to trip up, and figure out how you can do better tomorrow.

This appendix gives you space to record your daily food intake and daily exercise, as well as a place for you to reflect on spiritual lessons you're learning along the way. The journals included here cover an eight-week period, which should give you a solid start. But choosing a healthy lifestyle is an ongoing process, so I recommend that you continue your journal beyond the eight weeks. Feel free to copy the food and exercise journal pages to use for additional weeks, or you can continue your records in a separate notebook.

The reflection section for each week corresponds to the eight steps I've laid out in the book. You may complete these in conjunction with the related chapter, or you may want to change the order, depending on the particular issue you are struggling with in a given week.

WEEK 1

## Food Journal

| DATE | BREAKFAST | LUNCH | DINNER | SNACK |
|------|-----------|-------|--------|-------|
|      |           |       |        |       |
|      |           |       |        |       |
|      |           |       |        |       |
|      |           |       |        |       |
|      |           |       |        |       |

| DATE | BREAKFAST | LUNCH | DINNER | SNACK |
|------|-----------|-------|--------|-------|
|      |           |       |        |       |
|      |           |       |        |       |

## Exercise Journal

| DATE | ACTIVITY | MINUTES/REPS |
|------|----------|--------------|
|      |          |              |
|      |          |              |
|      |          |              |
|      |          |              |
|      |          |              |
|      |          |              |

## Reflection Journal

### STEP 1: Own Your Own Weight

What is the "weight" you are carrying? Why do you think it's difficult for you to take responsibility for this area of your life?

What's something you can do today to come clean and be honest—with yourself, with a friend, and with God?

Starting something new can feel both daunting and full of hope at times. As you begin your journey toward a healthy body and lifestyle, what feels most challenging to you? What feels most promising? Take a moment to reflect on Isaiah 43:18-19.

WEEK 2

## Food Journal

| DATE | BREAKFAST | LUNCH | DINNER | SNACK |
|------|-----------|-------|--------|-------|
|      |           |       |        |       |
|      |           |       |        |       |
|      |           |       |        |       |
|      |           |       |        |       |
|      |           |       |        |       |

| DATE | BREAKFAST | LUNCH | DINNER | SNACK |
|------|-----------|-------|--------|-------|
|      |           |       |        |       |
|      |           |       |        |       |

## Exercise Journal

| DATE | ACTIVITY | MINUTES/REPS |
|------|----------|--------------|
|      |          |              |
|      |          |              |
|      |          |              |
|      |          |              |
|      |          |              |
|      |          |              |

## Reflection Journal

### Step 2: See God as Your Friend

How do you see God? What lies have you believed about Him?

Based on God's true character, what are some things that would be His will for your life?

The second week into your journey, what are some things you are starting to learn about yourself? What have you been discovering about other people and about God? Read and reflect on Romans 8:31-38.

WEEK 3

## Food Journal

| DATE | BREAKFAST | LUNCH | DINNER | SNACK |
|------|-----------|-------|--------|-------|
|      |           |       |        |       |
|      |           |       |        |       |
|      |           |       |        |       |
|      |           |       |        |       |
|      |           |       |        |       |

| DATE | BREAKFAST | LUNCH | DINNER | SNACK |
|------|-----------|-------|--------|-------|
|      |           |       |        |       |
|      |           |       |        |       |

## Exercise Journal

| DATE | ACTIVITY | MINUTES/REPS |
|------|----------|--------------|
|      |          |              |
|      |          |              |
|      |          |              |
|      |          |              |
|      |          |              |
|      |          |              |

## Reflection Journal

### STEP 3: Take Up a New Perspective

Can you think of times in the past when God has used a difficult situation for a higher purpose? What are some purposes God might have in mind for the struggle you're going through right now?

What are some specific ways you can change your perspective about the issue you're struggling with?

How has your perspective begun to change since you took on the challenge to "start somewhere"? Look at Romans 8:18-28 and consider God's perspective on the difficulties you face.

WEEK 4

## Food Journal

| DATE | BREAKFAST | LUNCH | DINNER | SNACK |
|------|-----------|-------|--------|-------|
|      |           |       |        |       |
|      |           |       |        |       |
|      |           |       |        |       |
|      |           |       |        |       |
|      |           |       |        |       |

| DATE | BREAKFAST | LUNCH | DINNER | SNACK |
|------|-----------|-------|--------|-------|
|      |           |       |        |       |
|      |           |       |        |       |

## Exercise Journal

| DATE | ACTIVITY | MINUTES/REPS |
|------|----------|--------------|
|      |          |              |
|      |          |              |
|      |          |              |
|      |          |              |
|      |          |              |
|      |          |              |

## Reflection Journal

### STEP 4: Get Someone to Hold You Accountable
What level of community do you have in your life now? Are there some areas in your life where you need more accountability?

Write down the names of several people who could hold you accountable—perhaps a mentor, a trainer, a pastor, or a friend. Commit to contacting them sometime this week and asking for their help.

Now that you've been working toward your goal for almost a month, how supportive have your friends been? Read Ecclesiastes 4:9-12, and ask God for the kind of support described in this passage.

## WEEK 5

## Food Journal

| DATE | BREAKFAST | LUNCH | DINNER | SNACK |
|------|-----------|-------|--------|-------|
|      |           |       |        |       |
|      |           |       |        |       |
|      |           |       |        |       |
|      |           |       |        |       |
|      |           |       |        |       |

| DATE | BREAKFAST | LUNCH | DINNER | SNACK |
|------|-----------|-------|--------|-------|
|      |           |       |        |       |
|      |           |       |        |       |

## Exercise Journal

| DATE | ACTIVITY | MINUTES/REPS |
|------|----------|--------------|
|      |          |              |
|      |          |              |
|      |          |              |
|      |          |              |
|      |          |              |
|      |          |              |

# Reflection Journal

## STEP 5: Start Somewhere

What goal do you want to accomplish? Write it down, and make a commitment to follow through on that decision.

List the baby steps that will be required to accomplish your goal.

What baby steps forward have you taken so far toward your goal? What steps have you taken backward? Read Isaiah 40:28-31 for encouragement when you feel like you can't keep going.

# WEEK 6

## Food Journal

| DATE | BREAKFAST | LUNCH | DINNER | SNACK |
|------|-----------|-------|--------|-------|
|      |           |       |        |       |
|      |           |       |        |       |
|      |           |       |        |       |
|      |           |       |        |       |
|      |           |       |        |       |

| DATE | BREAKFAST | LUNCH | DINNER | SNACK |
|------|-----------|-------|--------|-------|
|      |           |       |        |       |
|      |           |       |        |       |

## Exercise Journal

| DATE | ACTIVITY | MINUTES/REPS |
|------|----------|--------------|
|      |          |              |
|      |          |              |
|      |          |              |
|      |          |              |
|      |          |              |
|      |          |              |

## Reflection Journal

### STEP 6: Eliminate the Excuses

What excuses do you frequently find yourself making? Who or what do you often blame for your failures?

What new habits can you start to replace your old negative patterns?

Now that it has been six weeks, what has surprised you so far? Is there anything that has been more difficult than you expected? Are there times when your response to a situation has been different from what it has been in the past? Read and reflect on 2 Corinthians 5:1-10.

WEEK 7

## Food Journal

| DATE | BREAKFAST | LUNCH | DINNER | SNACK |
|------|-----------|-------|--------|-------|
|      |           |       |        |       |
|      |           |       |        |       |
|      |           |       |        |       |
|      |           |       |        |       |
|      |           |       |        |       |

| DATE | BREAKFAST | LUNCH | DINNER | SNACK |
|------|-----------|-------|--------|-------|
|      |           |       |        |       |
|      |           |       |        |       |

## Exercise Journal

| DATE | ACTIVITY | MINUTES/REPS |
|------|----------|--------------|
|      |          |              |
|      |          |              |
|      |          |              |
|      |          |              |
|      |          |              |
|      |          |              |

## Reflection Journal

### STEP 7: Accept the Need for Training Wheels
In what situations do you find it most difficult to surrender to God's will?

Think about the specific triggers that tend to hold you back from God's best for you. Who or what will serve as your training wheels in those areas?

As you look back over the past seven weeks, what changes have you seen in yourself? What progress do you take most satisfaction in? What setbacks have been most discouraging? Read Joshua 1:6-9 and consider God's willingness to help you fight your battles.

WEEK 8

## Food Journal

| DATE | BREAKFAST | LUNCH | DINNER | SNACK |
|------|-----------|-------|--------|-------|
|      |           |       |        |       |
|      |           |       |        |       |
|      |           |       |        |       |
|      |           |       |        |       |
|      |           |       |        |       |

| DATE | BREAKFAST | LUNCH | DINNER | SNACK |
|------|-----------|-------|--------|-------|
|      |           |       |        |       |
|      |           |       |        |       |

## Exercise Journal

| DATE | ACTIVITY | MINUTES/REPS |
|------|----------|--------------|
|      |          |              |
|      |          |              |
|      |          |              |
|      |          |              |
|      |          |              |
|      |          |              |

## Reflection Journal

### Step 8: Persevere to the End
What obstacles have been most daunting for you in your journey toward wholeness? Have you noticed a pattern about when you get discouraged?

What truths can you hold on to when the miracle feels far away?

As Jeff said, "Losing the second 50 pounds is harder than losing the first 50. . . . The second 100 will be harder than the first 100. The closer you get to your goal, the more grit you will need." If you are feeling discouraged because progress seems slow, don't give up. Read Philippians 3:10-14 and journal about what it will mean for you to forget the past and press on to what lies ahead.

- <u>Patches</u>

Lidoderm
Lidocaine
Patch 5%
- up to 3 patchs
  a day
- can leave on
  12 hrs